Praise For Norman Shealy & Dawson Church's
Soul Medicine

"Soul Medicine is the perfect prescription for the healthcare crisis that is currently undermining our civilization. In their compelling synthesis, Norm Shealy and Dawson Church skillfully interweave ancient wisdom, spiritual healing, and leading edge science in defining a credible foundation for the emerging practice of energy medicine. This book is a must read for patients and professionals who are perplexed with the current state of healthcare."

—Bruce Lipton, Ph.D.
Cell biologist and best-selling author of The Biology of Belief

"Everyone should read this powerful book and compelling book. It is a most credible effort to examine the future of modern medicine, as it rediscovers the subtle energies of emotions, beliefs, and spirit. Soul Medicine bursts with astonishing research by pioneers, whose work deserves validation in tightly controlled experiments, critically reviewed, undertaken by scientists of the highest caliber. If replicated, they offer possibilities as revolutionary for medicine as if visitors came to Earth from another dimension, carrying advanced knowledge. Modest, humble, reasonable—and yet full of important truths—this book supports the importance of soul medicine becoming a treatment modality as routine as established specialities."

—Tom Stern, M.D.
Coauthor of The Heart of Healing *and other books*

"To indigenous peoples, 'medicine' has always been based on soul or spirit. In contemporary culture, the concept of mind-body medicine has gained wide acceptance. It is now time to seriously incorporate the third leg of the healing triangle: the soul. This well-written and comprehensive book invites us into this greater realm of healing or soul 'medicine.'"

—Ann Nunley, Ph.D.
Provost Emeritus of Holos University, author of Inner Counselor

"Jesus taught the importance of the faith of a mustard seed and demonstrated that faith in healing. In their very fine book Soul Medicine, Dawson Church and Norm Shealy explore the science behind such a faith and its many practical uses for our modern lives."

—Alan Davidson, CMT
Author of Spirit Living Through Your Body

"There is no shortage of adventurers in the realms of exploration, finance and politics. Finding true 'adventurers in ideas' is more of a challenge. We must welcome and applaud this collaboration between Shealy and Church for they are both adventurers in ideas that enhance and empower the life of the body and of the spirit. Soul Medicine is a fine and timely book."

—Ralph Blum
Best-selling author of The Book of Runes

"Soul Medicine paints the big picture of spirituality and healing as no book before, and a vast and gorgeous picture it is. Church and Sheely are visionaries whose far-ranging scope will inspire healing artists and the men and women of medicine for many years to come.

—Geralyn Gendreau, MFT
Coauthor of Healing Our Planet, Healing Our Selves

"In the art and science of healing, there are many paths up the mountain. While the goal of the summit may be the same, the paths are varied. In Soul Medicine, Norm Shealy and Dawson Church provide us not with just a map of the terrain, but a complete travel guide including history, path choices, scenery, traveling companions and potential difficulties and pitfalls. A masterful work, and entertaining to boot!"

—David E. Miller D.C.
The People's Chiropractor

"Having been a psychotherapist and international seminar leader for over twenty-five years, I finally was able to satisfy my need to understand how energy healing works. While deeply intrigued about alternative forms of physical, emotional, mental and spiritual healing, I had remained somewhat skeptical about the use of 'invisible forces' working with patients. My traditional training did not offer me any basis from which to comprehend the phenomena of energy healing.

"This book describes a coherent set of principles involved in the energy healing process. It offers a larger perspective and overview of the different alternative treatment modalities and bridges the gap between traditional approaches and the quantum paradigm of healing. This book makes enormous sense to read for anybody, who has been intuitively drawn to alternative healing approaches but was afraid to be led into speculative and unproven therapies.

"This book uncovers the beliefs inherent in our Western disease-centered paradigm and offers a comprehensive overview of alternative treatment approaches. It provides a cognitive map to make sense of the healing power of invisible energies. It opens the door to a quantum model for healing and gently invites you to cross over the bridge and rethink the process of healing."

—Gabriele Hilberg
Psychotherapist and Business Consultant

"Future generations, looking back, will regard conventional medicine during the twentieth century as being as limited as five-finger arithmetic. A new medicine is arising—one which embraces spirituality and consciousness as emphatically as conventional medicine has dismissed them. For a look at this medicine of the future, Norm Shealy and Dawson Church's Soul Medicine is invaluable."

—Larry Dossey, M.D.
Author of The Extraordinary Healing Power of Ordinary Things

Soul Medicine

Awakening Your Inner Blueprint for Abundant Health and Energy

C. Norman Shealy, M.D., Ph.D.
Dawson Church, Ph.D.

www.SoulMedicineInstitute.com

Elite Books
Santa Rosa, CA 95403
www.EliteBooks.biz

Library of Congress Cataloging-in-Publication Data

Shealy, C. Norman, 1932-, Church, Dawson, 1956-
Soul Medicine: awakening your inner blueprint for abundant health and energy /
C. Norman Shealy & Dawson Church. -- 1st ed.

  p. cm.
Includes bibliographical references and index.
ISBN 0-9710888-8-8
1. Alternative medicine. 2. Mind and body. 3. Soul--Health aspects. 4. Health--Religious
aspects. 5. Spirituality--Health aspects.
I. Dawson, Church. II. Title.

R733.S534 2006
610--dc22

2006001830

© 2006 C. Norman Shealy & Dawson Church

Portions of several chapters in this book were first published in *Sacred Healing* © 1999
C. Norman Shealy. The tables in Chapter Seven were originally published by, and are
copyright © Dr. Marcus Bach and the Fellowship for Spiritual Understanding and are
reproduced by kind permission of Mrs. Marcus Bach.

The information in this book is not to be used treat or diagnose any particular disease
or any particular patient. Neither the authors nor the publisher is engaged in rendering
professional advice or services to the individual reader. The ideas, procedures and
suggestions in this book are not intended as a substitute for consultation with a
professional health care provider. Neither the authors nor the publisher shall be liable or
responsible for any loss or damage arising from any information or suggestion in this book.

Typeset in Mona Lisa and Hoefler Text
Printed in USA
First Edition

10 9 8 7 6 5 4 3 2 1

This book is dedicated to everyone in the healing arts. Throughout history, those souls who have seen the suffering around them, and resolved to make a difference through their own lives, have been shining examples of the finest divine qualities in humanity.

Contents

Section I

The Trail of Miraculous Cures

Section II

The Soul's Historical Primacy in Healing

Section III

Quantum Healing

Section IV

Energy, Electricity and Therapy

Section V

Soul Medicine of the Future

Foreword
Caroline Myss, Ph.D.

Healing, by definition, is a sacred art. Practically all of the ancient texts describe the art of healing as a divine process in which healing the body first requires healing the spirit. When the potential of technical and chemical medicine accelerated during the second half of this century, the "spirit" of healing was made ill. That is, the consciousness that healing is a sacred art was eclipsed by a more scientific modality. Though not a deliberate intention on the part of the scientific community, respect for the healing power of prayer, faith and love diminished dramatically as chemical medicine produced more and more physical results.

The one of these three internal qualities that retained a position of respect within the allopathic medical community was faith. Even then, the energy of faith had to be directed toward supporting the potential healing technologies of the allopathic community. The healing power of faith was reduced to a personal matter that carried little or no authority in the external world. It seemed that, as the scientific and medical community accelerated in its growth and development, faith became a property of a more religious arena.

The entry of the scientific mind into the medical world has been and remains essential. The research done in these past five decades has been a masterful contribution to the knowledge we need to have about the chemistry and physiology of our own bodies. But somewhere along the line, the precious role of the Sacred has been reduced to the status of superstition and non-provable thought, dropped completely from the list of significant factors that contribute to health or the disintegration of health.

This book, *Soul Medicine,* looks at the interior of the human soul and honors its position of power within the human body. The authors lead the reader into the history of sacred healing, beginning with the ancient Romans and Greeks. This journey examines the role of religion and religious rituals that revolve around healing as well as the sacred sites that emerged during that time. They also introduce the reader to contemporary sacred healing and the research that has been done to study the effects of sacred techniques such as prayer and the laying on of hands.

The authors of *Soul Medicine* draw together numerous angles into one unified pattern, presenting an insightful view of the challenges that the contemporary healer faces within our culture. From an initial search for authentic healers that began in 1972, exploring various cultures and spiritual traditions, the authors have gathered an encyclopedia unto itself. This incredible book is a product of over three decades of experience with gifted healers—and reports on their successes and failures.

I have personally known Norm since 1984. While I recognize that he is a brilliant physician, I think of him first as the quintessential research scientist whose primary interest in this life is to discover more about the relationship of the energy—or sacred texture of the human being—to the physical body. Dawson Church has amassed an incredible breadth and depth of experience in the field of holistic and integrative medicine. This is their life's passion, and this passion is evident in every page of this book. They have thoroughly investigated, and continue to investigate, alternative sacred healing techniques, the foundation of soul medicine. In this book, they share years of personally investigating some of the most prominent energy healers of our time, describing their techniques and their successes. They knew (and know) many of these healers, and they write about them with clarity and discernment.

For all of us who are interested in understanding the nature of healing, this book is a necessary part of our library. It is becoming increasingly evident that the themes of this next millennium are healing and the emergence of the sacred into the entire weave of life. Norm Shealy and Dawson Church have performed a valuable service in presenting Soul Medicine.

—Caroline M. Myss, Ph.D.

Acknowledgments

We are deeply grateful to the following peer reviewers who offered us their comments on draft copies of the manuscript:

Ralph Blum

Larry Dossey, M.D.

Geralyn Gendreau, MFT.

Gabriele Hilberg, Ph.D.

Jeanne House, M.A.

David Miller, D.C.

Caroline Myss, Ph.D.

Ann Nunley, Ph.D.

Bob Nunley, Ph.D.

Tom Stern, M.D.

We also acknowledge the many healing professionals who we have met, whose work and words have inspired us. We are especially grateful to those who helped us with our research, or made us aware of studies and techniques that made their way into this book. We are also grateful to our families for giving us the support, love, and quiet space to work on the manuscript, especially Angela Church and Jeanne House.

SECTION I

The Trail of
Miraculous Cures

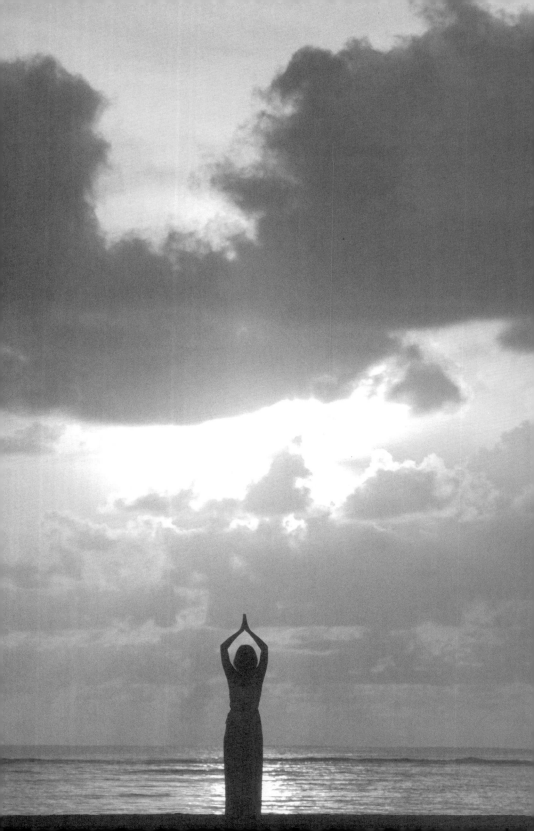

1

The Convergence of Spirit and Science

"**M**ichelle, a bright, perky, 21-year-old woman, arrived in my office complaining of severe bladder pain. She had to urinate frequently and urgently. I did a complete medical workup but could find nothing out of the ordinary—by the standards of my profession there was nothing wrong with Michelle. Yet it was clear to me that Michelle's pain was real, and her physical symptoms were real. After I had finished looking in her bladder with a cystoscope and found everything to be normal, I ventured, 'Sometimes women with your symptoms have a history of sexual abuse or molestation. Is this possible with you?' In the corner of her eye, the slightest of tears welled up. It turned out that Michelle had been sexually penetrated by an uncle almost daily from the age of three, till she was ten years old.

"I asked Michelle to think back upon these memories and find a part of her body where they were strongest. She said she could feel them acutely in her lower abdomen and pelvis. I asked her to rate them on a scale of 1 to 10, with 1 being the mildest and 10 being the most intense. Michelle rated her feelings at 10 out of a possible 10.

13

"I then spent 45 minutes working with Michelle, using some simple yet powerful emotional release techniques. I then asked her to rate her level of discomfort. It was a 1—complete peace. I urged her to cast around in her body for the remnants of any of the disturbed feelings she had previously felt. She could not find them, no matter how hard she tried. The emotionally charged memories had been so thoroughly released that a physical shift had occurred in her body. Her bladder condition disappeared. In the three years since that office visit, it has never once returned."

This account was written by Eric Robins, M.D., a urologist working at a Kaiser Permanente hospital in California.[1] It is one of thousands of similar stories of physical healing brought about by non-physical means. As well as a vast body of anecdotal evidence, an enormous and growing number of scientific studies now validates the principles of spiritual healing. Twenty years ago, a book entitled *Soul Medicine* would have been a metaphysical treatise. Today, it represents the cutting edge of scientific discovery, as you will see in the pages to come. Sacred healing, for centuries the domain of mystics, priests and charlatans, is today attracting some of the brightest and most innovative scientific researchers on the planet.

The revolution that their research studies is producing is overturning some of the most firmly established principles in the scientific firmament. Take the notion that the characteristics of our fifty-trillion-celled human bodies are produced by blueprints in our DNA. This idea is so firmly rooted in both popular culture and scientific literature that almost every week we read about this gene being linked to that behavior or that gene being linked to this trait. "Scientists today announced they have found a gene for dyslexia. It's a gene on chromosome six called DCDC2," announced National Public Radio on October 28th, 2005. The following day, the *New York Times* carried a long story of the same discovery under the byline "Findings Support That [Dyslexia] Disorder Is Genetic." Other US media echoed the story. Arch-establishment doctor, Stephen Barrett, M.D. summed up the prevailing view with the words, "some diseases are an inevitable result of genetic make-up."[2]

In fact, the entire notion that our destiny is written into the code of our DNA is crumbling. In his groundbreaking new bestseller *The Biology of Belief,* Bruce Lipton, Ph.D., points out that human beings have about 25,000 genes. Chimpanzees have a similar number. A lowly marine worm, *Caenorhabditis elegans,* each example of which has just 969 cells (one half-trillionth of the number found in a human being) has 24,000 genes. When the human genome project started, researchers were expecting to find at least 120,000 genes. That's how many they projected it would take to provide the blueprint for an organism as complex as a human being. They found just 23,688 genes—around one-fifth the expected number.[3]

If the information to build a human body, and create as magnificently complex a structure as the human mind and emotional realm, is not found in the genes, where does it come from? What is organizing structures as elaborate as the neural system and behavioral predilections? The answer must lie in a source of information beyond the genes, and science is just beginning to grapple with the awesome implications of these questions.

The new discipline of *epigenetics* looks at the influences on DNA from outside the cell. It is beginning to show that the biochemical environment in which cells exist has a profound effect upon which genes are activated. And the energy environment has an even more rapid effect than the chemical one on gene function. The journal *Science,* in a special 2001 issue of the magazine devoted to this emerging discipline, defined epigenetics as: "the study of heritable changes in gene function that occur without a change in the DNA sequence."[4] The old view of genes—one that still dominates science and the media—is that genes determine physical characteristics, disease propensity, and many behaviors. The new view, in the words of Karl Maret, M.D., is that "the genome is plastic and resembles constantly rewritten software code rather than being fixed hardware that you inherit at birth."[5]

In a quantum universe, space and time are probabilities rather than absolutes. The science of physics was shaken to its core a century ago by the emergence of quantum physics. When the first discoveries of quantum physics were made, and its implications began to reverberate throughout research and theory, the certainties of the old Newtonian physics were overthrown. Medicine today is in the grip of a similar revolution. Bruce Lipton says, "Conventional medicine works with the iron filings, whereas a deeper form of healing would attempt to influence the magnetic field. Most doctors don't see the field, so they're trying to figure out the relationship between the filings without even trying to incorporate the energy field in which they exist."[6]

In a Newtonian universe, the healing agents—drugs, doctors, surgery, hospitals, healers, shamans—must be present in the same space and time as the patient in order for healing to take place. In a quantum universe, the energy field in which a patient exists can produce healing without any need for a spatial or temporal connection. Phenomena like distant healing—healing across great distances, or even across time—are conceivable. A quantum universe is a set of probabilities, susceptible to influence by many factors, including thought, will and intention. It is a universe in which spontaneous remission of disease is possible, and in which the influence of a healer using non-physical means can be as effective as conventional medical treatment.

"The picture most people call 'scientific' is obsolete," according to quantum physicist Ervin Lazlo. He tells us that science is in the midst of "a shift from matter to energy as the primary reality" and that, "In the emerging concept of the new sciences there is no categorical divide between the physical world, the living world, and the world of mind and consciousness. Matter is vanishing as a fundamental feature of reality, retreating before energy; and continuous fields are replacing discrete particles as the basic elements of an energy-bathed universe."[7] In later chapters, we will examine in great detail some of the great spiritual healers of our time, and of history, and see what their methods and experience can contribute to our understanding of the energy universe in which healing takes place. We will also look at the lessons from cell biology, quantum physics, and brain physiology that shed light on the biophysical mechanisms at work in soul healing. Physicist Sir James Jeans said, "the stream of knowledge is heading towards a non-mechanical reality; the universe begins to look more like a great thought than a great machine."[8]

Lipton's experiments illuminate in great detail the mechanisms by which the membranes of cells change in order to admit or deny entry to certain proteins, which in turn activate genes. The activities of the mind, he shows, affect body functions, and changes in thinking and belief can have a direct effect on our cells. "When someone has a sudden shift of belief," he states, "it can radically change the epigenetics, which means that the same genetic code will now be interpreted completely differently—this could be the difference between cancer and remission."[9] He notes that the existence of these mechanisms shows why conventional medicine, alternative therapies and energy medicine can all be effective in producing healing. Each of them may be affecting the field through their own method of intervention; as the field changes, the patterns of iron filings change right along with it. In the words of researcher James Oschman: "In the past it had been thought that the genes give rise to proteins that then spontaneously assemble into the living structures that carry out living processes, including consciousness. In the emerging quantum model, it is the action of quantum coherence that organizes the parts into living structures, and it is the action of quantum coherence that gives rise to consciousness as a distributed and emergent property of the assembled parts."[10]

Soul medicine makes medical use of that quantum coherence that gives rise to consciousness in order to effect healing. It harnesses the healing power of consciousness, regardless whether that consciousness is expressed through alternative medicine or conventional medicine. Soul medicine does not deny or negate conventional medicine. The last six decades of biomedical and pharmacological research have managed almost completely to overlook the study of such crucial factors in healing as consciousness, electromagnetism, faith and prayer, and quantum processes. Soul medicine simply restores these factors to the equation.

One study examined 442 patients at the Baptist Family Practice clinic in Morrow, Georgia. It used several different in-depth tests to determine how healthy they were overall, how much pain they were in, and how strong their intrinsic spirituality was. The results of the various tests were then compared, to determine whether or not there was a correlation between spirituality and wellness. The researchers found that the patients with the strongest intrinsic spirituality had the least pain, and were healthiest overall.[11]

A group of researchers from St. Luke's Medical Center in Chicago looked at the link between church attendance and physical health. It found that those with a regular spiritual practice were more likely to be healthy and had a lower mortality rate.[12] Another similar study at the University of Texas Medical School led by Thomas Oxman examined the effects of spiritual or religious practice and social support on people undergoing heart surgery. Their findings revealed that patients who possessed a large and deep social network, or were devoted to their religious or spiritual practice, exhibited just *one-seventh* the mortality rate of those who did not.[13] Another recent study found that patients prayed for had "six-month death and re-hospitalization rates about 30 percent lower than did control patients."[14] Results as astonishing as these are far from being the exception. They are the norm. Larry Dossey, M.D., author of *Prayer is Good Medicine*[15] and other similar books, points out that there are upwards of 1,200 studies that explore the interface between health, longevity, and religious and spiritual practices, with more in progress.[16]

A fascinating series of experiments on the effect of consciousness on the structure of the DNA molecule has been performed by the Institute of Heartmath in Boulder Creek, California, led by Rollin McCraty, Ph.D. The researchers there took DNA samples drawn from human placental tissue, and measured changes in the protein's structure when exposed to the *intentions* of individuals. They used spectrography to measure the degree of twist in the double helix of the DNA molecules in the samples. This characteristic can be determined by measuring the degree of absorption of ultraviolet light exhibited by the DNA molecule.

Experimental samples of DNA were then exposed to human intentions. Groups of individuals were asked to hold the intention that the helixes of the DNA in the samples would twist tighter. In other experiments, they were asked to intend that the spirals became looser. The samples were then tested to see if there was a measurable change, in the desired direction, looser or tighter.

Untrained volunteers were unable to have any effect on the degree of twist in the DNA molecules. The samples measured the same before and after they were exposed. Even trained individuals from the Institute staff were unable to have any effect using will and intention alone.

However, those same people then entered a calm, meditative, state that the Heartmath researchers call "heart coherence," because the heartbeat is unusually regular in this state. When they held an intention while in a state of heart coherence, the structure of the DNA samples did indeed change. When samples subject to the thoughts of volunteers who held the intention of the DNA twist becoming tighter were later examined, the molecules were found to have a tighter twist. In some samples, the degree of twist had increased by an astonishing 25 percent, a huge effect. When subjects entered the appropriate mental and emotional state, then held the intention of the DNA unwinding, the twist was found to have loosened. The researchers then repeated the experiment at a distance, to control for any possible influence from the electromagnetic fields of the volunteers' hearts, brains and other organs. Even at a distance of fifty miles, the effect was replicated.

One highly trained volunteer, able to achieve an extremely stable state of heart coherence, was found to be particularly effective at changing the twist in DNA molecules. In one experiment, three separate vials of placental DNA were prepared, A, B and C. He was asked to tighten the degree of twist in A and C, but not in vial B. When the ultraviolet characteristics of the DNA in all three samples were later examined, the result was exactly as he had intended, with an increased twist in vials A and C, but no change to the molecules in vial B. This suggests that, far from producing a generalized effect, intention is highly specific.

McCraty and his team of researchers conclude that: "the data presented here support the concept that cell-level processes can be influenced by human intention, mediated via energetic interactions." They also suspect that these positive mental and emotional states might be implicated in many other aspects of energy medicine, in spontaneous remissions, and in the placebo effect, as well as in the documented value of faith and prayer in improving health and longevity.[17] They demonstrate that by focusing directly on soul healing, we may produce positive changes in our physical condition.

The implications of such research are stunning. They show that by changing our consciousness, we can change the very blueprints around which our physical bodies are constructed. We can first seek healing close to the source, by intervening in our own thinking, rather than trying to deal—much later on down the line—with the ill effects of our thoughts on our bodies. While it is unlikely that we will ever be able to bypass physical means like drugs and surgery for the healing of every disease in every person, these new insights show clearly that soul medicine is the very first intervention point we should look to for physical or emotional healing. It's free. It's not under the control of an HMO, doctor, hospital, or spouse. It usually feels good to great. It places awesome power over our own healing within us. It returns the responsibility for our well-being to our own doorsteps, rather than displacing that responsibility onto some outside agent of healing. And research is screaming at us with the urgent message that consciousness can harness the powerful healing forces of a quantum universe, forces far more potent than pills in a bottle.

In past generations, spiritual healing was perceived as a mystical, otherworldly event. To many people, and some scientists, it still is. It's like old maps of the New World. The shape of the coastline in one of the first maps of America, produced by Spanish cartographer Diego

Gutiérrez in 1562, and now reposing in the Library of Congress, is so close to reality that if you put it side by side with a modern atlas, all the key features are recognizable. But when it came to interior detail, the cartographers could provide only clues and guesses. This is where our understanding of spiritual healing lies today. While experiments like the ones described above tell us clearly that consciousness affects DNA, we are still a long way from being able to say that *this* thought held simultaneously with *that* feeling produces *this* effect. We know the general outlines, but not the details. "If at first the idea is not absurd," observed Albert Einstein, "then there is no hope for it."

Former neurosurgeon Norm Shealy, M.D., Ph.D., one of the two coauthors of this book, met Olga Worrall, one of the most famous healers of the twentieth century, in the early 1970s. At that time, she conducted healing services every Thursday morning at the Mount Washington United Methodist Church in Baltimore, Maryland. There were about three hundred people at each service. She stated that the healing service "just exhilarates me. I feel seven feet tall. I'm just a channel for the healing power, but the power comes from spiritual sources, not from me." She had some *fifteen thousand* letters in her possession from grateful recipients of healing. Norm was able to obtain medical records for ten patients. These showed "miraculous" healing that defies medical experience.

Another master healer Norm evaluated was a "Persian" (he refused to use the word Iran) named Ostad Hadi Parvarandeh. Ostad graduated from the American University in Tehran and eventually became a diplomatic counsel to France. Over the next few decades, he served in a number of countries, including Greece, Yugoslavia and Bulgaria, before retiring in 1976. Soon his home became a clinic. At times, so many people gathered outside the house requesting his attention that police had to assist with traffic control. As a result of treating so many people, he became well acquainted with medical terminology. He also began to document his cases in an effort to pass his knowledge on to others.

Norm set out to find out if any of the accounts of healing were genuine, verifiable medical cures. He asked patients for permission to contact their doctors, and eventually obtained the medical records of 100 patients. Here are some of those accounts, written by medical professionals, for which Norm has medical documentation:

An M.D. ophthalmologist writes in January 1996, "Mr. Suarez been my patient since 1986 and was under my supervision. His vision gradually was lost due to macular degeneration in both eyes so that he was not able to drive. At present his vision is improved after visiting Mr. Parvarandeh, and he is able to drive because of improving vision in both eyes."

A psychologist and director of a major pain clinic wrote to Ostad, in March 1996: "I have been quite amazed by the progress shown by several of my patients who have seen you."

A New York M.D. wrote to Ostad, in March 1996, "I was profoundly impressed with your capability to provide significant and documented—need I say almost miraculous—benefit to a large variety of often very difficult cases in the face of prior unsuccessful attempts by the best Western medicine has to offer."

A Philadelphia scientist wrote to him in March 1996 as follows: "We were amazed at your extraordinary capacity to diagnose rapidly and treat patients with subtle energy and the power of intention in our presence, some of whom have lasting pain relief or other improved conditions as a direct result of your treatment. Everyone I spoke with following your visit here is greatly impressed with your abilities."

A board certified M.D. family physician wrote in 1996, "I have witnessed the healing of illnesses that go far beyond the capacity of conventional Western medicine."

A doctor of Oriental Medicine wrote in July 1996 that his son had had serious problems with Crohn's disease for five years, with frequent diarrhea; he had lost 40 lbs. Initially Ostad treated the son over the phone for five minutes. Immediately the diarrhea ceased and the pain was less severe. After the second and final treatment, "symptoms dramatically decreased. He began tolerating normal foods, and over the next four months totally stopped taking all medications and gained thirty-eight pounds."

A doctor of Oriental Medicine and acupuncture wrote that he had observed Ostad "greatly improve and cure the ailments of different patients such as cancer, incurable viruses, seizures and even blindness, and the Master has not only cured his patients, but has also rejuvenated the life back into their spirits." He said that even manic depression and schizophrenia have been no challenge for Ostad Parvarandeh.

A New Jersey physician wrote, "I witnessed the effect of his healing power on several patients." He then goes on to describe eight of them:

1. The first patient was a fifty-eight year old doctor who underwent spinal fusion surgery in 1987 and developed paralysis of the right lower limb due to complication of surgery, later confirmed by MRI examinations. The surgeons were not interested in further surgery. After his first therapeutic session with Ostad, a very fine movement was noted in his right toes. After forty sessions of therapy, the patient, who had been paralyzed, could walk with a walker and crutches, and is currently practicing medicine in his office. I'm not aware of any nonsurgical intervention or therapy that could ameliorate such organic spinal cord injuries in such a short period of time.

2. A thirty-two-year-old woman, the wife of a doctor, developed amenorrhea and galactorrhea, which persisted four years after giving birth to her second child. The patient was treated by Mr. Parvarandeh for three sessions. Her symptoms disappeared and her menstrual cycles were normal. In the first session the patient was seen in person by Mr. Parvarandeh, and the next two sessions were done over the phone.

3. A thirty-five-year-old woman, the wife of a doctor, developed a severe frontal throbbing headache. In spite of all physical examinations and laboratory and paraclinical tests such as MRI and

CT scans, no definite cause was identified. Ophthalmologic exams were normal. It was diagnosed as a nervous headache, and she used painkillers. Mr. Parvarandeh diagnosed the headache as being due to minimal liver dysfunction. It is noteworthy that all liver function tests were within normal range. After a few sessions of therapy in which Mr. Parvarandeh was concentrating on her liver, the headache disappeared. This is a new idea not known by medical doctors that liver dysfunction, even in the presence of normal function tests, could exist and lead to headache; it is believed there is no known medication for such treatment.

4. After transfer of energy to the liver of several patients with hypercholesterolemia and hypertriglyceridemia by Mr. Parvarandeh, the blood levels of triglycerides and cholesterol dropped significantly. There was no medication that could do the same.

5. A sixty-seven-year-old surgeon who has liver cirrhosis developed thrombocytopenia. After receiving the healing energy of Mr. Parvarandeh, platelets increased from 20,000 to 50,000 and the size of the spleen decreased.

6. I have also witnessed the decrease of chest pain in patients with proven angina pectoris and myocardial infarction.

7. A patient with frozen shoulder, after fracture of the head of the humerus, regained full function of the shoulder joint after a few sessions of therapy with by Mr. Parvarandeh.

8. A five year-old girl was diagnosed with alveolar soft part sarcoma of the right leg in 1986. The tumor showed histological evidence of muscular and vascular invasion. Pathological diagnosis was confirmed at a center in England and in the United States. The patient was referred to a center in England where she received a course of chemotherapy, and she was discharged with a diagnosis of metastatic sarcoma to the lung with no further therapy. She has since then been under treatment by healing power of Mr. Parvarandeh and is still alive and doing well 10 years after the initial diagnosis. This case is one of the very rare long-term survivals of metastatic sarcoma,

and may be the only case of long-term survival in metastatic sarcoma of the lung.

We know from stories like this that something is happening. We can't clearly articulate how and why it happens—yet. As our experimental data on spiritual healing increases, we are discovering that its effects are vast. The dozens of scientific experiments on the effect of consciousness upon physical healing show, time after time, that spiritual practice and belief have a marked positive influence on longevity and health. They have been found to:

- improve the survival rate of patients after operations,[18]

- ameliorate pain,[19]

- raise levels of pleasure-inducing hormones in the brain,[20]

- improve mental acuity,[21]

- reduce depression,[22, 23]

- boost immune system function,[24, 25]

- reduce the time it takes wounds to heal,[26]

- reduce the frequency and length of hospital stays,[27, 28]

- increase marital happiness in men,[29]

- reduce alcohol consumption and cigarette smoking,[30, 31]

- reduce the incidence of cancer and heart disease,[32]

- improve the health of older adults,[33, 34] and

- add years to the average life-span.[35, 36]

What phenomenon is at work here? Science can confidently correlate a vibrant spiritual life with all kinds of healing effects. Science can study individuals like Olga Worrall, Ostad Parvarandeh and the many others you will be meeting in the pages of this book. Science can identify and measure magnetic, electrical, and other subtle energy fields which are being affected by sacred healing. Science can catalog the many vehicles by which sacred healing takes place, from visits to shrines like Lourdes, to prayer, to acupuncture, to massage. What science has a great deal more trouble with is putting them all into a unifying big picture, and explaining where the epigenetic control comes from that produces these miraculous cures. That's where the concept of soul healing comes in.

What will the trajectory of our developing knowledge of soul medicine look like?

Imagine a circle of Neolithic men huddled around a fire pit. In the center, there is a pile of kindling and logs, ready to burn. One man, dressed in skins and feathers, with a bone necklace and skin pouches hung around his neck, has special knowledge: the fire-starter. With a primitive bow, he rapidly rotates a hard stick against a piece of soft wood. Both are carefully positioned against a ball of dry moss. After much rubbing, the hardwood shaft produces a tiny spark. The fire-starter wraps the moss around the spark and starts blowing gently through his fingers.

At first, nothing happens. Then a puff of smoke comes from the center of the moss. Then heavy gray smoke starts pouring through the fire-starters fingers. A tongue of flame shoots upward, and the fire-starter thrusts the burning moss into the center of the kindling. All the men gathered around him gasp, then cheer, as the flames leap upward in the dark night, striving for the stars.

To early humans, the process seemed like magic. Only a few initiates possessed the esoteric knowledge of how to start a fire. It might have seemed like a gift from the gods, a supreme shamanic mystery, an occult ability to summon a spark of the sun to warm the night.

Today, we know the physics of every step of the process. Anyone can be taught to be a fire-starter. Today we have maps of the interior, as well as of the coastline.

Our knowledge of soul medicine is still at the stage that mapmaker Diego Gutiérrez was in 1562. We know the rough shape of what the effects look like. We have the effects produced by healers like Olga Worrall and Ostad Parvarandeh to guide us, as well as thousands of accounts of spontaneous remission from patients.

We have instruments capable of measuring the human energy field to tolerances impossible a century ago. But we are still far from understanding the mechanisms that produce these effects. Further research over the course of the next few decades will allow us to map the interior as well, and reduce what seems like an esoteric mystery to a well-charted series of procedures. Science, which for so long dismissed the entire realm of soul medicine as superstition or anecdote, is now the engine pushing our understanding of its principles to new levels of precision.

We are entering a new era of healing. Soul medicine, like fire-making, is no longer a mystery guarded by shamans. It is being investigated, described, cataloged, and understood by science. The gifts of soul medicine are on their way toward becoming a routine part of medical treatment, just as Dr. Robins was able to treat Michele at his Kaiser Permanente hospital practice, and clear up a long-standing medical problem using energy medicine. Dr. Robins is an example of the new kind of physician. While he practices as a conventional urologist in a large urban hospital, he is not afraid to step beyond the boundaries of his discipline when looking for cures for his patients.

Yet though they may become routine, these techniques will never lose their wonder. The mystery endures. Last month, at a men's retreat, the group sat in a circle. The men were drawn from all walks of life; there were cooks, computer technicians, corporate CEOs, mechanics, ministers. We still gasped when one of our number stood up tall, held a ball of flaming moss to the heavens, and made a fire.

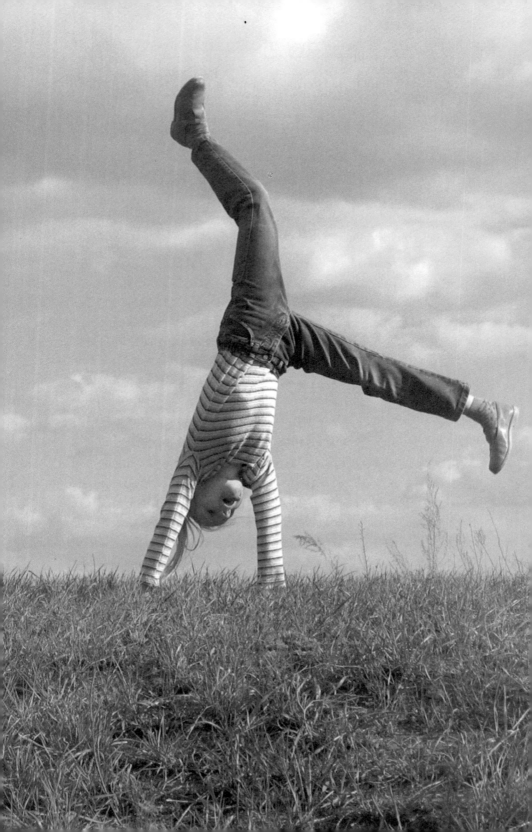

2

The Blueprint of Perfect Health

The experience of having an eternal living soul has been part of human conviction from antiquity. In the 1940s, Carl Jung, the great Swiss psychiatrist, studied people around the world and reported that approximately 90 percent of individuals—in virtually all cultures—believe in

- life after death (a soul);
- a supreme being (God);
- the Golden Rule (treat thy neighbor as thyself).

The soul may be thought of as a personalized expression of the universal field, as the divine aspect of a human being, of God expressed at the level of a single being, or as personhood made manifest through pure consciousness, as opposed to physical or mental form.

Jung stated that people who do not share the age-old beliefs listed above do not thrive. We believe that an existential crisis of doubt about purpose or spiritual meaning in life is a major root cause of many illnesses. Soul connection promotes health, and obstructions to soul connection promote disease.

For a person who embraces the sacred as the foundation for all life, the physical body is primarily a mechanism for soul expression on the physical level. It is consciousness—and its links with spirit or soul, and through that with God—that has the capability to convey the sacred to the material world. Human consciousness can reflect the qualities and intentions of soul consciousness. When human consciousness does not reflect and transmit the qualities and powers of that soul, we discover that significant psychological and physical illness can result.

Modern medicine began to forget the power of sacred healing centuries ago, and embarked on a materially focused healing path. The sacred aspect of human beings has been largely ignored by medicine ever since. Allopathic medical practice does not account for the link between healing, the soul, and God. Yet studies and experiments are increasingly challenging this mechanistic model, and providing us with hard empirical evidence of effects of soul medicine that conflict with purely mechanistic explanations of how life works.

Study of the mechanism of a piano will reveal very little about the nature of sound. The music of the piano will reveal little of the nature of the consciousness of the pianist. A study of the automobile will reveal a bit about the nature of metal and engines but nothing about the driver or the engineers who designed the car. Likewise, the study of the physical body in itself reveals nothing specific about the nature of the spirit or the divine or the sacred. Yet the pragmatic experience of many practitioners from many healing specialties reveals that we are endowed with tremendous resources within to heal both physical and emotional problems.

Doctors, science writers, and researchers have danced around the concept of the soul for a generation. We've been prepared to document the *correlation* between spirituality and health, but we've been reluctant to stick our necks out and wonder what's actually *causing* all these health effects. It's one thing to summarize research indicating a *link* between belief and healing, and quite another to *ascribe* healing to the thing believed in. In *Soul Medicine,* we examine the overwhelming evidence for sacred healing. We list the many forms through which it flows. We look at some of the remarkable physical mechanisms that link the spiritual and material aspects of human beings. We assume the existence of the soul. And we also take the next great leap, arguing that if there is a soul, it can express abundantly through the body, mind and emotional realm of each person. It is also our personal experience that healing flows through this soul connection, and that removing blocks to this flow promotes health. The connection between soul and body is made through consciousness, actuated by intention; changes in consciousness trigger changes in health.

The Three Pillars of Soul Medicine

The premise of soul medicine is this: *We allow the perfect consciousness of health contained in the soul to express freely in the patient's energy system. Through this intention, healing is triggered in heart, mind, and body.*

Soul medicine rests on three pillars. The first is the concept of the human being as an *energy system.* Healing is approached at the level of the energy system first, not at the level of the presenting condition. Illnesses, diseases and symptoms are respected. They are considered as valuable guides, prompting both healer and patient to notice energy imbalances and correct them. They are sources of information, rather than simply nuisances to be made to vanish. Energy systems are matrices of connection; a change in any one part changes the whole, and a change in the whole rearranges the parts. A change in the energy field works itself outward into physical change, and can clear a symptom.

Essentially, everything in the universe as we understand it is energy. Every atom in the body vibrates at a certain energy level. Collectively, each of us has a unique individual "energy signature." We are all electromagnetic entities. Our soul has a field of a certain vibrational frequency, as we will discover when we delve deeply into the subject of electromagnetism and healing. When we consciously bring our minds and hearts to a similar vibration, so that they are functioning in the same vibrational range as our soul, then there is resonance between them, and reciprocal communication between their energies. This allows healing to flow effortlessly through to the body.

There is abundant experimental evidence that there are many currents of energy coursing through each human body. They are responsible for the health of all the major systems, and organs. They control the regeneration of cells, the development of the fetus, the speed of recovery from disease, the expression of certain genes, and many vital functions.

We cannot measure the soul in the same way we measure a material phenomenon, yet we are beginning to be able to measure some of ways in which energy shifts during soul healings. Highly intuitive individuals from all cultures have been able tune into this dimension for millennia. They see energy in and around human bodies. Science is now mapping many of the phenomena which they have been able to perceive. Ervin Lazlo reminds us that, "The shift in science's view of the world is reflected already in the most fundamental notions we have of reality: matter and space... In the emerging concept there is no 'absolute matter,' only an absolute matter-generating energy field. Space-time... is a virtual-energy medium that can be perturbed—one that can create patterns and waves. Light and sound are traveling waves in this continuous energy field, and tables and trees, rocks and swallows, and other seemingly solid objects are standing waves in it."[1] Soul medicine seeks to perturb the virtual energy of space-time in the direction of health, and to measure the changes in energy fields produced by this perturbation.

Consciousness: The Second Pillar

The second pillar of soul medicine is *consciousness*. Energy systems are affected by consciousness. A change of consciousness automatically changes the energy system. Consciousness is the first place to turn when seeking healing.

Consciousness is implicit throughout the universe, and our souls connect our local selves to that greater consciousness. Consciousness connects us to the quantum field in which all things are possible. Physicist Arthur Eddington observed: "the stuff of the world is mind-stuff... The mind-stuff is not spread in space and time... Recognizing that the physical world is entirely abstract and without 'actuality' apart from its linkage to consciousness, we restore consciousness to the fundamental position."[2] Soul medicine restores consciousness to its rightful position at the forefront of healing. The conscious person notices the many potential outcomes present in the field, and by intention, nudges the field in the direction of the highest possible outcome. When human consciousness holds a strong intention of being one with divine consciousness, allowing itself to be conditioned by the consciousness of the soul, then the enormously expanded range of possibilities present in soul awareness, including miraculous healings, become possible. The reality picture of the soul becomes the reality picture of the body.

The work of faith healers provides a living example of the healing effects of consciousness. Their awareness appears to be unbounded by the limits of consciousness of most of humankind, and they seem to be able to transmit that healing faith to those that seek their touch. Faith healing has been with us since the dawn of time; a miraculous cure that usually occurs through the laying on of hands, originally by kings or priests, but in modern times by a number of religious and spiritually oriented practitioners. Kathryn Kuhlman, Ostad Parvarandeh, and—the most studied of all—Ambrose and Olga Worrall, are but a few of these modern healers. We have learned much by analyzing them, and discovering how energy flows during their treatments. Yet it has pointed us inevitably toward recognizing that while these miracle healers are particularly adept at channeling energy, there is something happening in their consciousness that sets them apart. They always ascribe their powers to God, and they invariably have strong spiritual practices or religious affiliations.

Even people who don't think of themselves as spiritual or

intuitive may experience soul consciousness during peak experiences. Peak experiences occur when the focus of our identity shifts from our bodies, our minds, and our circumstances—the mire of *thinking*—to the realm of pure awareness, unmediated by thought. Meditators seek this experience on a daily basis; mystics in every moment. In an ecstatic spiritual state consciousness in which the boundaries of personal and eternal dissolved, the poet Rumi exclaimed:

> A secret turning in us
> Makes the universe turn![3]

Such is the conscious experience of being one with soul. In this state, the distinctions between one's own personal soul, and the universal soul, vanish. Your participation in the experience of your own soul makes you one with the experience of all soul. Individualized soul is thus our gateway to the experience of universal soul. David Fagerberg, a Catholic theologian at the University of Notre Dame, observes that, "'The human being is microcosmic.' Being a microcosm of God, he said, 'does not mean a fraction of the whole, it means that everything in the whole can be found here in a smaller scale.'"[4] During peak meditative and healing experiences, the experiencer sees only the perfection of that macrocosm. Perceptions of limitation, whether they be physical disease, confinement, emotional turmoil, doubt, worry, or anxiety, all fall away. They are replaced by a state of pervasive peace, and a sense that all is well.

This is the consciousness in which the medicine of the soul may flow into the body. It draws on the power of the universal soul, particularized in the individual soul, to promote healing. It connects with the epigenetic blueprint of healing available at the soul level; at that level, all healing is possible, even miraculous cures. By identifying with that soul level, and the blueprint for health contained at that level, the image of greater perfection can migrate into the concrete physical reality of one's mind, heart, and body.

Even when a person does not have the faith to gain access to the perfect blueprint of health contained at the soul level, they may be healed by contact with a healer who does have that faith. A healer may see the perfection inherent at the universal level, having the consciousness that, "God sees John as perfect"—and by the strength of his or her conviction, midwife the perfection of the soul's healing power into a diseased body. A patient's faith—even in a surgeon or pharmacist—is an enormous portion of the cure. As Jesus said, "Thy faith has made thee whole."

Intention: The Third Pillar

The third pillar of soul medicine is *intention*. Affecting energy, projected into the field of consciousness, intention is what shapes a healing outcome. Without intention, the potential in the field of consciousness remains untapped. The healer engages that latent potential through the power of intention. A master healer is able to hold intention even when the patient's intention has broken down. Weak or conflicted intentions can never be as effective at producing healing as strong and unambiguous intentions.

Intention provides the power, the motive force, to set in motion the complex chain of events that results in healing. The potential for a cure may have been present in a patient's genome before a visit to a master healer, but it is not set in motion until the healer's intention begins to condition the patient's energy field. All the ingredients were there in the field, and the recipe of health was available in the form of a genetic blueprint. Then, the healer's intention provides the organizing principle around which the healing event takes place. Intention conditions the field of consciousness, reorganizing energy into the configuration required for healing.

The intent of our soul is that our body be healthy. At the soul level, we have access to healing wisdom, and the infinite knowledge of the Great Soul, the accumulated wisdom of the quantum field of infinite possibilities. There are healing possibilities in this infinite field that are completely beyond the borders of our present knowledge. When we still our busy minds, and attune our experience to the vibration of the soul, we have access to those healing possibilities. Intention then trips the switch to put them into concrete expression as wellness.

35

Healers are people who have become adept at attuning their personal energy fields to the imprints of health present in the infinite field, and holding a powerful intention for healing in another. When a sick person enters the field of a healer, and is infected by the healer's intention, their field is conditioned by that of the healer and reorganized, producing an effect different from that produced by the sick person. Yet the field exists independent of a particular healer, and, with intention, can be accessed by any of us. The mind itself, we are discovering, can transcend time and space, and enter realms in which time as we know it does not exist. These capacities have seemed mysterious, yet science is now catching up; very recent research is beginning to provide us with an outline of some of the processes at work in soul medicine. Healing—mediated by *consciousness,* and activated by *intention*—occurs when the patient's *energy system* is triggered to conform to the soul's blueprint.

The Many Faces of Soul Medicine

Many therapies facilitate soul healing. The method that you use to connect with the consciousness of perfection contained in your soul is less important than the fact of connection. It is making the connection that allows healing to flow. Many therapies—perhaps all therapies—make the connection. Even drugs and surgery may have their most powerful effects by stimulating the patient's belief system. In later chapters we will review some of the hundreds of research studies showing that most of the results of drugs and surgery are attributable to patients' belief in their efficacy. Drugs and surgery, where they are effective, may derive most of their effectiveness from soul medicine, the engagement of the patient's conscious belief system. Edgar Cayce observed that, "Perhaps, in reality, the doctor, psychologist, and priest are the workers at the same laboratory table, the molders of the same ductile clay, three tenders of the same divine fire."[5]

Soul medicine seeks to safely remove the blocks and barriers to the flow of energy through our systems according to that soul blueprint, whether those blocks be spiritual, physical, mental, emotional, or energetic. The concept of soul medicine ties together many consciousness- and energy-based therapeutic healing modalities. Therapies that put us in touch with that soul connection are all part of the field of soul medicine. They include many of the modalities grouped together as "complementary and alternative medicine," or CAM, as well as prayer, healing touch, and faith healing. Some of those we will delve into in subsequent pages are:

- Acupuncture, acupressure, shiatsu, meridian tapping, and other therapies based on the body's energy meridian system

- Aromatherapy and essential oils

- Physical manipulation, such as osteopathic and chiropractic adjustments, massage, and other somatic therapies

- Meditation, contemplation, retreats, and other techniques for calming the mind

- Electromagnetic stimulation

- Laying on of hands, Therapeutic Touch, Reiki, Attunement, and other non-touch energy transmission modalities

- Prayer, and Faith Healing by a bona fide healer

- Light and color therapies

- Homeopathy and flower essences

- Biofeedback and creative visualization

- Conscious Lifestyle, including conscious exercise (stretching, dance, yoga, martial arts, or any exercise done deliberately) conscious eating, and other healthy lifestyle changes

- Traditional medical practices such as Shamanism, Ayurveda, and Oriental Medicine

- Affirmations, muscle testing, and other therapies that influence the subconscious mind

Soul medicine is a unifying concept that explains why so many different therapies work. By fostering the understanding that human beings are energy systems, it tells us that whenever some portion of the energy field is affected by a treatment, the entire system is affected. An intervention at any one point affects the whole energy body. Professor Helen Graham of Keele University writes, "These new conceptions of reality require bodies, health and disease to be viewed as dynamic processes rather than discrete entities, and understood in terms of patterns of relationships with the organism and its environment rather than in terms of separate parts."[6]

A treatment that promotes the free flow of energy, or an increase in energy at some point, is an effective treatment. Soul medicine is a collection of treatments that remove energy blockages and permit the free flow of energy. Which treatment is used depends on what is most effective for that condition or that patient. Any of the above modalities can be effective at promoting increased energy flow. Soul medicine is not invested in any one modality; it is invested in increasing the energy flow in the whole system. Soul medicine does not favor Ayurveda over chiropractic, or biofeedback over prayer. It recognizes that certain modalities work well for certain conditions, and that some patients are more responsive to a particular therapy than another.

As a conceptual approach to healing, soul medicine is invaluable. By focusing on the energy system as a whole, and by portraying treatment as a means to increasing energy flow, it simultaneously explains how many different treatments can be effective, and seeks to pinpoint the particular therapy that provides the most powerful leverage point for each patient's energy system.

Energy Healing as Primary Care

Soul medicine consciously focuses on therapies without negative side effects. Rather than going first to metabolism-altering drugs and risky surgical procedures, you can open up the vast natural pharmacopoeia of your body by engaging the positive beliefs and intentions that reside in soul consciousness. Safe and non-invasive procedures like prayer, energy healing, acupuncture, lifestyle change, electromagnetic stimulation, and the others on this list, are much safer than drugs and surgery—and have none of the miles-long list of side effects associated with many of them. Soul medicine is the first step in responsible medical treatment.

Soul medicine redirects the focus of healing away from symptoms, and away from a focus on the outer manifestations of disease. It focuses on the spiritual connection between the soul and body, and seeks to remove blockages to the free flow of energy between soul and body. It operates on the assumption that removing those blockages and allowing a free flow of energy will have an effect on the symptoms, and open the door for "miraculous" cures such as the ones described above. The therapies in this list all have the potential to remove such blockages and open the gates of energy to permit healing.

While a concept such as soul medicine would have been a metaphysical curiosity a generation ago, today it is on the leading edge of scientific research. In this book, we reference hundreds of scientific studies that point to the link between spirituality and healing, between energy therapies and healing, between beliefs and intentions and healing, between prayer and healing, and between faith and healing. Some were performed a century ago; some were published just days before this book went to press. The evidence is piling so high that it is impossible to ignore. We also examine some of the thousands of accounts of miraculous cures that occur in the course of soul medicine.

Yet for all the weight of research quoted in this book, our scientific understanding of soul medicine is at its infancy. We believe that medicine is on the threshold of an explosion of new research into the links between spirit and body that will illuminate the mechanisms by which healing takes place. The reason for this research interest is that the effects of soul medicine on healing can be enormous, often far more dramatic than the best drug or surgery available. As the research studies pile ever higher, they are stimulating a revolution in the practice of medicine and healing that ripples through every corner of the world.

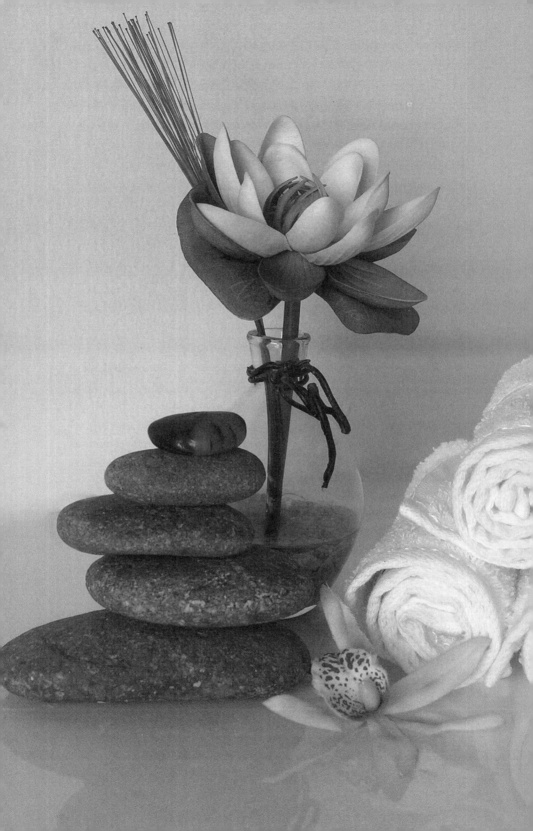

3

A Physician's Search for Sacred Healing

NORMAN SHEALY, M.D., PH.D.

I have always known that there is a universal power we generally call "God," as well as an aspect of us, the soul, that survives physical death.

Although my family was only minimally attached to the concept of going to church, I found the church's rituals comforting and attended regularly throughout my childhood and early adolescence. I grew up attending a Southern Methodist church that was remarkably liberal for its day. Teenagers were allowed to dance on Sunday evenings in the basement of the church. I was not aware of the teachings of guilt that seem so prevalent in many religions today. In my mid-teens I was on a statewide debating team taking the positive side of the debate, "And God so loved the world that He gave His only begotten son that whosoever should believeth in Him would not perish but have everlasting life."

At age sixteen I went off to Duke University where I was often inspired by the sermons of Dr. McClellan, a wonderful Presbyterian minister. Then at nineteen, I entered medical school, three years younger than most of my classmates. I had little time for religion or even thoughts of spirituality over the next eleven years as I pursued medical school, internship, and ultimately a neurosurgical residency at Massachusetts General Hospital. Halfway through the neurosurgical residency, I became engaged, and my fiancée and I discussed at length our spiritual beliefs and what church we would attend. We settled on Trinity Episcopal in Boston, primarily because Dr. Theodore Ferris was one of the most charismatic ministers I've ever encountered. We attended couples' discussion groups at his home about once a month, whenever my schedule allowed.

During post-residency I was still busier with neuro-surgery and raising a family than I was with spiritual and religious activity. In October 1971, I founded the first comprehensive pain clinic in the United States. I was dealing with people for whom conventional allopathic medicine had failed. Many of them had undergone multiple, unsuccessful operations. In fact, my average patient had gone through five to seven unsuccessful back operations. Many of them were much worse neurologically and experienced more pain than before the first operation.

In 1972 a synchronous series of events took place. The most important, perhaps, was meeting Olga Worrall, whose work will be discussed at some length later in this book. I had been invited to speak at Stanford University to a group of 1,200 physicians on the value of acupuncture; at that conference I met Olga. I also met Dr. Bill McGarey and subsequently was introduced to the teachings of Edgar Cayce.

Olga and I instantly became friends and remained so for the next thirteen years, throughout the remainder of her life. Through Olga, I was introduced to the concept of "sacred healing." Yes, I was aware that Oral Roberts apparently talked about doing healing on his radio and television programs. My grandmother had been a great fan of his. I was vaguely aware of Katherine Kuhlman and her work in healing. Yet Olga got my attention partly because she had been scientifically studied, and those studies confirmed many unusual abilities and reports of near-miraculous healing.

Knowing how difficult it is to heal many illnesses, especially through neurosurgery, I became fascinated with the idea that miraculous sacred healing could occur. I visited Olga at the Mt. Washington United Methodist Church in Baltimore, where each Thursday morning about three hundred people attended her healing service at the New Life Clinic.

At the end of August 1972, I visited the Association for Research and Enlightenment (A.R.E.) in Virginia Beach, which houses the Edgar Cayce readings. Edgar Cayce is best known as the "Sleeping Prophet" who did almost 15,000 trance "readings," about two-thirds of them related to illness and healing. "The Week of Attunement," as the conference was called, changed my life even further. Twice I had what is often described as a peak experience, a literal awareness of my connectedness with God and the universe.

Those two events, meeting Olga and the Week of Attunement, led me to the principles and experiences of autogenic training and meditation and finally to a quest for the essence of spirituality. I began collecting letters to Olga from people who claimed she had healed them. Through them I attempted to collect medical documentation to prove sacred healing had occurred as described in these letters. Interestingly, even with the patients' permission, few physicians answered my requests for medical records.

One of my most profound experiences occurred when I was a senior resident of neurosurgery at the Massachusetts General Hospital. One evening, a man brought his comatose sister into the hospital emergency room. An emergency X-ray of the arteries to the brain demonstrated a moderate tumor in the right frontal lobe, and I removed that tumor, which turned out to be a metastatic squamous cell carcinoma. The woman recovered consciousness overnight. The primary cancer was found to be an exquisitely small tumor in the urethra, and it was apparently cured with radiation.

During the days after her recovery, however, she was extremely agitated and weepy, and one day I said, "If you do not improve your attitude, you will never get well." She replied, "Oh, Dr. Shealy, are you a Christian Scientist, too?" Her agitation had to do with the fact that she had failed to cure herself and had succumbed to medical treatment, including surgery. I explained to her that I considered all aspects of healing, including medical and surgical therapy, to be God-given.

In 1975 I was invited to debate Dr. William Nolen, a surgeon and popular author, on "The Tomorrow Show" with Tom Snyder. Dr. Nolen had written a book titled *Healing: A Doctor in Search of a Miracle.* Dr. Nolen properly emphasized that healers such as Katherine Kuhlman seemed to feel that many of their cures took place through "the holy spirit." He asserted that many of the illnesses may have been psychosomatic and the results purely the power of suggestion or "placebo."

One case reported in Dr. Nolen's book, however, infuriated me. I knew the patient; he had a pituitary tumor and had lost his ability to see out to the side from either eye. He had been in a hospital in San Francisco and was so distraught after the neurosurgeon there told him all the risks of surgery that he walked out of the hospital in the middle of the night. He went to the Philippines to have "psychic surgery." Two years later, he had totally normal visual fields and no symptoms whatsoever. Dr. Nolen's book, however, gave a different history of this case. On the air I told Dr. Nolen that I thought he had deliberately distorted the facts.

Despite his relatively negative approach toward sacred healing, Dr. Nolen admitted that a significant majority of patients, perhaps as many as 70 percent, were improved by spiritual healers. Yet he concluded his book with "Healers can't cure organic diseases. Physicians can." Then he went on to say, "So let us admit that healers do relieve symptoms and may even, as I've already mentioned, cure some functional diseases." He adds, "We may well admit this; it's a fact—they're going to achieve an overall cure rate of 70 percent."[1]

Dr. Nolen's greatest conflict with the sacred healing issue apparently arose from within separate parts of himself!

His statement that he had been "unable to find any such miracle worker"[2] who could cure an incurable illness set me on a course to prove that miraculous healing truly occurred. Over the ensuing years I have reviewed more than one hundred medical records documenting miraculous cures. One white crow proves that there are white crows; we now have a huge flock of them. Sacred healing is alive and well.

The Next Step: Holistic Healing

In the meantime, the Shealy Institute that I founded in 1971 continued to work with patients with a wide variety of illnesses. A quarter-century after its founding, the American Academy of Pain Management, the largest organization of clinical pain practitioners in the world, reported that the Shealy Institute has the best success of any pain clinic they have evaluated—at a cost that is 60 percent lower than the national average. Our cost effectiveness in dealing with chronic pain of almost every type has been gratifying. When back pain is due to a ruptured disk, we can achieve better and safer results in 85 percent of patients than can be done with surgery. And for those with degenerative joints in the back, 75 percent of the time we can achieve similar results. 76 percent of patients with headaches have a marked reduction in both the frequency and severity of their headaches. This is almost twice as good as any drug on the market. We can get 85 percent of people out of depression with two weeks, safely and without drugs. This also is approximately twice as effective as any antidepressant and without any of the serious side effects. Currently I am training physicians and Nurse Practitioners to carry on this work as I think it may be the biggest contribution we can make to happiness and health.

Yet, what can be done for the 15 percent to 20 percent of patients who continue to have chronic pain? And for the patients who come to us with much more serious illnesses, such as cancer? Statistics published in 1997 in the *New England Journal of Medicine* appear to demonstrate that chemotherapy at best might add a few months of longevity to patients with breast cancer, but the quality of life is often markedly diminished.

Another effective healing method needs to be available, especially for those patients with medically and surgically incurable illnesses, and those who cannot be cured by the best of alternative medicine.

Soul medicine is that method. In this book, we present many summaries of cases of documented miraculous healing. We demonstrate the physiological effects of sacred healing, including changes in electroencephalogram (EEG), changes in the molecular bonding in water, and other effects, even on bacteria and enzymes.

I had long envisioned a graduate program where students would contribute meaningful research to the field of spiritual healing. In 2000 I collaborated with Drs Ann and Bob Nunley to establish Holos University Graduate Seminary. The seminary offers distance learning graduate, post-graduate, and certificate programs with selected residency requirements. Courses and research explore the emerging integration of historical, theological, and scientific foundations for optimal physical, mental, and spiritual health.

Holos amplifies the research dealing with spiritually-based holistic healing. It emphasizes ecumenical spiritual approaches that fulfill a growing need for the practice of soul medicine in contemporary communities. As a seminary, Holos places special emphasis on the spiritual aspects of its wellness studies and research. As a university, Holos strives to uphold the highest standards of excellence in teaching and scientific research and seeks to serve as a bridge between primarily academic institutions and primarily religious institutions. Holos course work demonstrates an appreciation for the essential teachings of the world's great religions and a broad ecumenical, interpersonal, and cross-cultural understanding of faith and spirituality. It supports a high degree of professional competency in holistically oriented spiritual counseling approaches, and independent scholarly study and research using rigorous protocols.

This holistic approach was a basic principle of the American Holistic Medical Association, which I founded in 1978. Soon thereafter the terms of *complementary, integral, quantum, integrative,* and *alternative* medicine became synonyms for holistic concepts of health care and well-being, and greatly extended the allopathic convention that has dominated American medicine for over a century. Acknowledging that most illnesses appear to have direct correlations with poor self-esteem, anxiety, and depression and, as such, may be rooted in an existential crisis of faith, Holos affirms the highest holistic and ecumenical spiritual principles as the foundation for optimal physical, emotional, mental, and spiritual health.

The Holos library website contains reference materials plus the abstracts and downloadable files of the theses and dissertations completed at the seminary. The seminary building in Missouri, completed in 2003, includes a spacious chapel, offices for the administrative staff, and classrooms for residency classes. Holos has already graduated over one hundred students with a doctorate in theology, with a focus on soul medicine. Holos graduates are accomplished spiritual and intuitive counselors.

In addition, Caroline Myss and I established the American Board of Scientific Medical Intuition, which certifies the competency of Medical Intuitives and Counseling Intuitives. As the institutions of soul medicine become formalized and defined over the course of the coming decades, training programs like that of Holos, and certification programs like that of the American Holistic Medical Association and the American Board of Scientific Medical Intuition, will play an increasing role in providing independent standards and public accountability for this emerging set of professions.

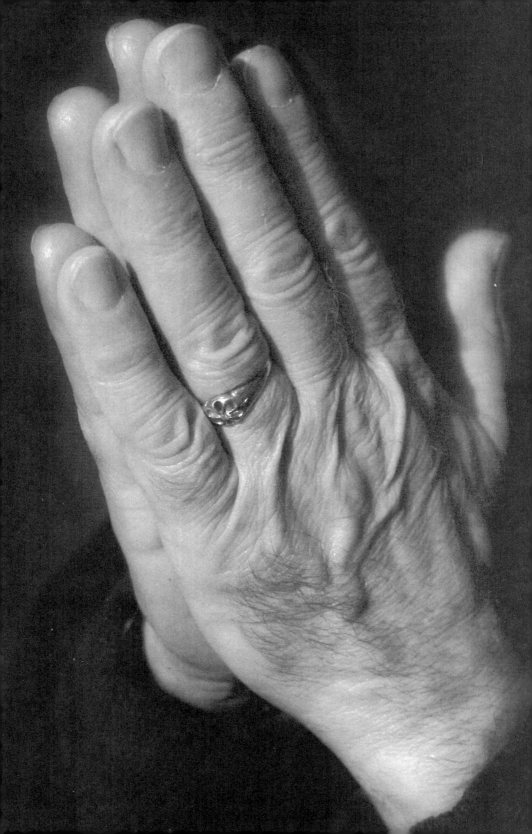

4

Magic Precedes Science

DAWSON CHURCH, PH.D.

I grew up, the son of a missionary Christian evangelist, in a home in which the church was central. My father was initially influenced by the Methodist church. He was ordained a Baptist minister, and eventually moved to the Charismatic Episcopal church, which combines Pentecostalism and Eucharistic worship. Yet in contrast to some anti-intellectual strains of Christianity I've encountered since, our family and social circle was anything but insular. We had more in common with the seventeenth and eighteenth century British clerics, intellectually curious, well-informed, and acutely aware of the social contexts in which their churches flourished. We discussed the issues of the day, political and religious.

For a minister in the nineteen fifties, church services happened on Wednesday night, Saturday night, Sunday morning (two services, maybe three), and Sunday night. That was on top of pastoral visits to the sick and dying, and a full schedule in the office. Parishioners came over to our house constantly—this was a society in which "dropping in" unannounced on the minister's home was a right every parishioner took for granted. In the course of my father's missions,

49

he and sometimes our whole family met many other ministers, of all denominations. Some of them were famous: Billy Graham, Nicky Cruz, Jimmy Swaggart, Richard Roberts.

The inevitable answer to every parishioner's or minister's problem—besides a cup of Earl Grey tea—was a prayer. The prayer was supplicatory, asking God to intervene in the healing of a sickness, the faltering of a congregation, the desertion of a spouse, or the loss of a job. One of my earliest memories, around the age of seven, was standing in a circle of praying men. It included my grandfather, my father, and an assortment of my many uncles (all of whom were ministers, priests, or deacons).

By that age, I was old enough to start noticing the enormous gap between what most ministers preached and how they lived. Seeing their behavior up close was a disappointment. I would watch a minister deliver an impassioned sermon on the love of Jesus on a Sunday, then belittle his wife, dismiss his children, and abuse his domestic servants on Monday. I became disillusioned with religion in general; if it truly had such transformative power, I wondered, how come its principles had so little effect on the daily thoughts and actions of its proponents?

The reason I remember that prayer circle so vividly is not the personalities of the men involved, or what they prayed about. I've long since forgotten the details. But when I closed my eyes, I noticed that there seemed to be a purple column of light and energy rising up from each man's head, that grew in intensity with the prayer. I remember furtively opening my eyes to see if this phenomenon was visible. With my eyes open, I could see nothing except a group of impassioned men, talking and swaying. When I closed my eyes again, there was the column again, with a turquoise haze around each purple column.

While our community was extremely religious, in terms of observance, it was not particularly spiritual, in the sense of an awareness of, and reverence for, the sacred. That came later, when I discovered the deep mystical tradition of Eastern Christianity, and the spiritual sophistication of Eastern religions, with their elaborate descriptions of subtle physiology, at the age of fifteen. Suddenly there was a place for the deep experiences of divine love that I had been having, experiences for which there was no echo in the fundamentalist Christianity in which I had been raised.

I began to take classes in the Perennial Philosophy at the heart of all religions. I also began to study sacred healing. The form to which I was first exposed is called "attunement." It resembles Therapeutic Touch and Reiki, except that the practitioner focuses on the body's endocrine glands. I noticed that an extremely strong current could be kinesthetically discerned when sharing or receiving an attunement.

I remember a particularly powerful experience of the power of attunement. My partner Brenda and I were working on a construction project. She was holding a window frame, while I was using a nail gun to shoot nails into the corners.

I pulled the trigger, and the nail I was shooting hit another nail already in the frame, deflected, and went right through Brenda's thumb, all in a split second. The nail went in through the ball of her thumb, and out the top through the middle of her thumbnail. The wound began to bleed profusely.

I sat down with Brenda, held my hands above and below her injured thumb, and began to use the basic attunement method, allowing a current of healing energy to flow between my hands. Before our eyes, the wound went through all the stages of healing. It stopped bleeding, then turned black and blue. As we held the current, the bruising went away. The shattered fragments of thumbnail knit together. Eventually, a little pink dot was all that remained in the middle of her thumbnail where the exit wound had been, along with another dot in the middle of the ball of her thumb where the nail had entered. The whole process had taken about twenty minutes. We went back to work.

When Brenda and I were expecting our first child, Lionel, I began to wonder if you could apply the attunement technique to a child in the womb. I noticed when I held my hands near pregnant mothers, I could feel the "energy signature" of the child—quite distinct from the mother's. Several times, I surprised women who had not told anyone they were pregnant, and had not yet begun to show, by asking questions about the pregnancy, after discerning a child's presence.

I found a strong current of connection with Lionel when I would hold my hands over Brenda's tummy. I began to share attunements with him almost every day, and a powerful bond began to grow between me and the baby. I wrote a book about these experiences called *Communing With the Spirit of Your Unborn Child,* in which I teach the basics of attunement in a form that can be used by any parent.

At that time, in the early 1980s, there was an almost complete split between conventional medicine (sometimes, quaintly termed "traditional" medicine, though of course there's nothing traditional about a medicine which ignores the spiritual aspects of healing) and "alternative" medicine. Chiropractors were shunned by the medical community, which regarded them as charlatans; the American Medical Association was still fighting in court to have the profession curbed. Acupuncture, visualization, and naturopathy were still regarded as dangerous quackery by most physicians. Materialistic medicine and spiritualistic medicine did not talk to one another.

Yet I sensed an inexorable flowing together of the streams. Nothing in soul medicine invalidates conventional medicine. Patients can get better using drugs and surgery, even while they're praying and using homeopathic remedies. Even the most ardent supporters of alternative medicine may take an aspirin for a headache. And conventional medical doctors who care deeply about their patients, as most of the finest ones do, are clearly connecting at a level beyond mere medical technique. True scientists are curious about new approaches, even when they violate the tenets of the current orthodoxy.

I first became aware of the pioneering work of my coauthor Norm Shealy when I was working on the 1984 Human Unity

Conference. That conference, and others sponsored by the Whole Health Institute, assembled together many figures prominent in the healing arts. In the late 1980s I published a collection of essays called *The Heart of the Healer.* It brought together surgeons, oncologists, chiropractors, acupuncturists, homeopaths, and vibrational healers in one volume. Because I assumed no rupture between alternative and conventional medicine, the book did not assume one either. It highlighted the elements common to all modalities, and was very well received and reviewed in the press.

I went on to distribute and edit many other books on healing, relationships and spirituality over the course of a long career in book publishing. I was inspired by many of the visionaries of our time, as the world shifted and the streams really did flow together. In 2003, the fifteenth anniversary of *The Heart of the Healer,* I edited a new anthology, *The Heart of Healing.* At that time, it was no longer necessary to argue strenuously that the streams were converging. It was an established fact. For several years, American patients had been spending more dollars, out of pocket, for alternative therapies than for conventional medicine. Doctors were looking to alternative therapies for answers, especially for chronic diseases that were intractable with conventional treatment. Alternative therapists were willing to recognize the limits of their efficacy, and refer patients to medical specialists when called for.

I have a strong bias toward science. I have encountered many self-styled "healers" whose methods seemed dubious and whose qualifications appeared murky. I would no more want one of them working on my subtle bodies than I would want an inexperienced or ungifted psychotherapist working on my psyche, or a medieval barber-surgeon sawing on my physical body. If soul medicine works, there must be good science that explains why. There are many phenomena in soul medicine that can not be explained by science—yet. This does not mean that they never will be. It simply means we do not yet have the experimental methods and designs to investigate them. As the experiments are developed and the theories tested, we are developing an increasingly sound scientific basis for soul medicine. We should not reject a miraculous healing phenomenon because science has not yet described the mechanisms behind it. And we should not reject science because its careful methods proceed at a pace that often lags behind the dynamic mystery of healing. "The scientist knows that in the history of ideas," observes Michael Gaugelin in *The Cosmic Clocks,* "magic always precedes science, that the intuition of phenomena anticipates their objective knowledge."[1] Larry Dossey, in his book *Healing Beyond the Body,* urges us to "Consider many therapies that are now commonplace, such as the use of aspirin, quinine, colchicine, and penicillin. For a long time we knew that they worked before we knew how.... This should alarm no one who has even a meager understanding of how medicine has progressed through the ages."[2]

I recently had an experience that illuminates many of the fault lines of contemporary healing. I was playing baseball at church camp, with a group of young men, in a lumpy meadow. I hit a home run, and began dashing around the bases as fast my long legs would carry me. In the same spot that had just laid low one of my teenage team mates, I tripped and fell spectacularly. Up in the air, then hard down on my left knee. I struck the ground with all 260 lbs of my body weight driving into the earth.

I knew right away that I had injured myself badly. I crawled to third base, then lay on my back in the dirt. I got up and tried to hobble off the field. My leg wouldn't support me, and friends helped me walk to a bench, and then to a camp bed.

The camp was in a remote area. One of the camp organizers asked me what I wanted. I knew there was an M.D. in the camp, who was also a vibrational healer, so I asked for her to be sent. Two Reiki practitioners, both, as it happened, Ph.D. biologists, were also handy. The three of them began working on me.

Ever since the moment I began falling, I had felt intensely present. I used this faculty for self-diagnosis. My knee was red, and had swelled up to the size of a football. I intuitively explored the tendons and muscles, wondering if any were torn. I wandered down the corridors of my body, noticing that my lower back and my neck both seemed to be out of alignment.

The physician-healer asked me all the right diagnostic questions. She touched my knee in various places; when she prodded on the left side of my kneecap, I screamed with pain. I didn't tell her about my back or neck, but she ignored my knee and began to work in those two places. She could sense, as well as I intuitively realized, that they were out of place, and that an energy correction to my knee would not hold unless they were aligned first. When she had done her work there, I felt a surge of energy all the way up and down my spine. She then moved her hands to my knee. With a big sigh, I went to sleep.

When I awoke, one of the Reiki practitioners was working at my feet and the other at my head. The doctor was holding her hands over my knee. It was still red, large and angry-looking. I winced at the slightest movement. A muscular friend half-carried me to the bathroom and back; I could not put the slightest pressure on my knee without almost passing out from the pain.

The camp counselor reappeared, and we all talked about the best thing for me. I did another intuitive scan of my body, and this time I was convinced that, despite the symptoms, nothing in my knee was torn or irretrievably damaged. I felt as though all I needed was rest and calm. I felt as though the healing process was well on its way.

No-one else in the room felt the same way. They wanted me to get to a hospital or emergency room as soon as possible. The nearest one was an hour's drive away. One practitioner thought I was being stubborn, and in denial about how serious the damage was to my knee, which indeed looked bad. The panic in the room at my resistance to leaving the camp was tangible. People were fearful of the consequences to the camp if a camper were injured and then not treated. With the consensus opinion being so strong, I felt as though it was very difficult to make my wishes heard. I wondered if these seasoned experts were right, and my inner sensing was no more than a delusion.

I eventually said, "Just give me another half hour of rest, and if my knee doesn't improve, I'll go to the hospital." My self-talk was, *If I don't heal this thing, and quick, these folks are going to make me leave whether I want to or not.* The other people went to arrange a four wheel drive jeep to get me across the trail to the nearest road.

With the room clear and still, I said to myself, "OK, now it's time for some rapid healing. I want the healing cycle to accelerate, and complete, now." I focused an intense beam of energy on my knee. My hands felt as though I had them in a fire. The air between hands and knee seemed to tingle, like the heat distortion above a flame. I pictured all the cells in my knee working harmoniously together to recreate themselves. I imagined all the healing resources of my body mobilized to assist my knee. The swelling began to go down. The redness began to diminish. I visualized torn tissue repairing itself at a frantic pace.

When my well-built friend came to assist me to the jeep, I got up and walked freely. There was little or no pain. There was still a little swelling, and a little redness. But the people who had seen me painfully attempting to hobble just half an hour earlier were amazed. They could hardly believe their eyes. I was walking proof that there was clearly no need for me to go to a hospital or emergency room. The jeep drove me back to my own cabin, where I rested for a little longer. Then I got up and resumed all the normal camp activities.

The next night was dance night at the camp. We had a hoedown, with a caller in a Western shirt and ten gallon hat singing out traditional square dances. I hopped and skipped higher than anyone else in the room. I checked in with my knee periodically, and felt a few twinges, but no warning signs. When the caller asked if we'd had enough dancing, I yelled, "No" and we made him keep going for another half hour. I was the last person to leave the dance floor, flushed, sweating, and happy as a clam. It was my own personal little celebration of the power of soul medicine.

I am not advocating that we abandon conventional treatments. Later in this book, we will look together in depth at which conditions conventional medicine excels at treating, and for which ones alternative medicine is best. But the body's innate self-healing mechanisms should always be the first place we look for healing. The body may require assistance in healing itself. That nudge might come from a Triple Warmer treatment by an acupuncturist, or the removal of a cancerous tumor by an oncologist. Either way, we can do no harm by adding the power of soul medicine to whatever treatment we choose. A few months ago, after I'd tried several alternative medicine cures for a blocked Eustachian tube, I went to my brilliant family doctor, Robert Dozor, M.D., who, after taking a careful case history, cheerfully wrote me a prescription for the strongest possible steroid suitable for the condition. Soul medicine, allied with the best of alternative and conventional medicine, is good medicine indeed.

The other day, my twelve-year-old daughter Angela had some radical dental work done. Afterwards, she took an aspirin, and a few hours later, another. But about an hour later, she said, "Daddy, the aspirin's not working, my mouth still hurts. Will you give me an attunement?" She's very much in the moment, and as she asked she lay down on the floor in the hallway, right where she had been standing! I held my hands over her, and her energy field responded very quickly. "How do you feel now?" I asked after about five minutes. "The pain's gone," she said cheerfully, and leapt to her feet.

I was incredulous, asking, "Completely gone?" She nodded, and raced away. My rational mind still has trouble reconciling itself to such immediate results—even when I see them right before my eyes.

The studies about DNA and consciousness that are described in Chapter One give us a start in understanding such effects. They also provide some of the missing links between conventional and alternative medicine. The implication of this research is that genes interact with consciousness, and consciousness with genes. The deeper I delved into this material, the more inspired I became to share this awareness with as many people as possible. I read books and studies voraciously, especially new experiments that shed light on the mechanisms of healing. I eventually wrapped my writing, practice and research into a dissertation. Norm Shealy was my dissertation committee chair, and when I read his book *Sacred Healing*, I proposed incorporating those ideas, plus current research, into this book.

These questions intrigue us both: How do miraculous cures, vibrational healing, electromagnetic healing, and traditional forms of medicine like Ayurveda, shamanism and acupuncture fit into the medical picture? What theory of healing explains the effectiveness of all of these practices? What is science telling us about the mechanisms behind healing? Which areas of healing are fruitful targets of future experimentation and study? What is the shape of a medicine that embodies the best of modern biomedicine, and the most effective practices of soul medicine? What will healing, hospitals and doctors look like to the next generation? This book contains some possible answers to these fascinating questions.

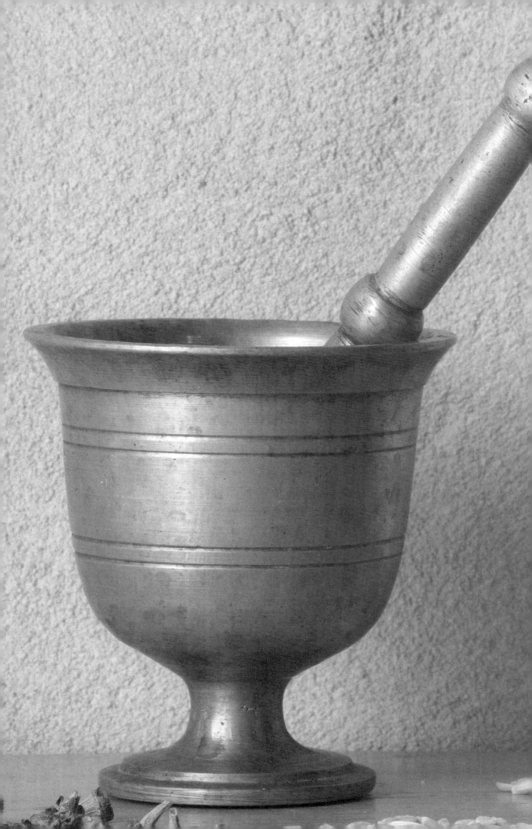

5

Outstanding Healers of Our Time

The vast majority of physicians go into medicine because of their compassion and altruistic desire to help patients. Most of them are healers in the true sense of the word. Yet they often wind up far from their goal, according to the *American Journal of Medicine,* which observed, "The current time-consuming training process often takes bright, creative young adults with a love for helping people, and turns them into cold, distant persons who have lost many of their original ideals regarding the practice of medicine...producing a physician with qualities 180 degrees opposite those it states it believes in."[1] Best selling author and physician Rachel Naomi Remen, M.D., writes, "Year after year, in medical schools across the country, the first-year class enters filled with a sense of privilege and excitement about becoming doctors. Four years later, this excitement has given way to cynicism and numbness. By graduation, students seem to have learned what they have come to do but forgotten why they have come."[2] Many genuine healers, like Ostad, don't even try, and instead choose the path of an independent healer. Here, free from the constraints of a disease-centered paradigm, they are able to do great good. "They simply 'know' they must become healers, and they will do almost anything to fulfill their calling.... Hearkening to a deep and primal drive..." says Larry Dossey.[3] Below, we look at some of these people, and their extraordinary healing abilities.

Harry Edwards, Foremost English Healer

Harry Edwards was perhaps the best-known sacred healer in England in the twentieth century, and former president of the UKs National Federation of Spiritual Healers. Due to his efforts to make faith healing an integral part of the medical repertoire, faith healers may have a formal position assisting with treatment in doctors' offices in England. He was undeterred by great hostility shown to his work by the British medical profession, and by the Church of England; those two bodies would not "admit that any other agency could achieve successful healings."[4]

He believed that anyone with a great passion and desire to help others could develop the ability to heal. Edwards said that the qualifications of a good healer include generosity, a willingness to give of self, compassion, and sympathy for those in need. He felt that individuals who want payment for their healing are too selfish and, therefore, not as likely to be outstanding healers.

After WWII, his healing practice came to national prominence, and by the mid-1970s, Edwards was receiving up to 9,000 letters a week from patients requesting absent healing. Though a gifted healer, Edwards believed that most people would have to return to him for treatment a number of times. A single healing experience rarely cured people of their disorders. He also encouraged patients to help themselves. In treating chronic arthritic conditions, for instance, Edwards recommended home massage and specific limbering exercises, in addition to multiple laying-on-of-hands sessions. He felt that a patient's mind has to be influenced in the direction of healing. Edwards believed that mental distress is caused by emotional and sexual problems, failure to attain one's ideals, and the desire of the inner self to express in a way that one's existing way of life might not permit. His assessment of his work was that 80 percent of his patients improved from his treatments and belief system; 30 percent were cured, and 10 percent were cured instantly.[5] He died in 1976, and his work is carried on today by the Harry Edwards Spiritual Healing Sanctuary at www.HarryEdwards.org.uk.

Olga Worrall: The Most Studied Healer of All Time

Olga and Ambrose Worrall conducted healing services at the Mount Washington United Methodist Church for almost thirty-five years. Olga continued the services on Thursdays after Ambrose's death. Norm was able to obtain the medical records of nine patients who had been miraculously cured by Olga of a variety of illnesses. Many attendees were repeat visitors; some wrote her grateful letters, for instance:

"During the service I felt heat moving throughout my body. My dizziness disappeared completely, and I have remained free of it now in the months since the healing service."

"My arthritis pain which had been virtually incapacitating for the last year has been almost totally absent since last Thursday morning. Praise God."

Dr. Elmer Green and his wife Alyce, psychology researchers from the Menninger Foundation, tested Olga Worrall. Their findings were most startling. They connected her to various pieces of electrical monitoring equipment, including an EEG, EKG, and skin galvanometer. She was placed in a room that had a vacant room on either side of it. Two more rooms along the hallway on the opposite sides of the vacant rooms were used. One was for recording the measurements during the study, the central control room. The other one, four rooms away, on the other side of the second vacant room, held the patient, wired in a similar way to Olga.

Olga could not see the patients she was treating, nor had she been introduced to them or informed about their problems. Her voice was recorded in the central control room, as were the devices monitoring both her and the patient. In four out of the twelve patients, there were striking simultaneous EEG changes associated with the exact moment during which Olga "sent" healing. When working with one patient, she stated, "I believe this patient smokes, as it feels as if I'm moving through molasses to get my energy to him." She was right; the patient was a smoker.[6]

Notable Contemporary Healers

Today there are many healers in the US who achieve remarkable results. This is not a complete list, but it includes several with whom we have had experience.

Rev. Ron Roth, a former Catholic priest, radiates joy in his work and lectures. Ron has many letters from patients who considered themselves healed. Norm obtained three proofs of miraculous healing from among this group. More case histories are reported in the book, *Healing Spirits* by Judith Joslow-Rodewald and Patricia West-Barker. Ron Roth emphasizes that psychological issues and spiritual wounds must be healed, in addition to physical ailments. He heads up Celebrating Life Ministries, where he works with many other people, including those of different faiths. He is the author of many books and a number of CDs and DVDs. His web site is www.RonRoth. com.

Michael Tamura is a spiritual teacher and healer. Over the course of more than three decades, he has assisted many in healing. He has written a book entitled *You Are the Answer;* his web site is www. MichaelTamura.com. He and his wife Rafaelle practice in Mount Shasta, California, and travel widely.

The work of Sister Justice Smith, a professor at Rosary Hill College in Buffalo, New York, has been of great importance. She found that Mr. Esterbane, a healer studied extensively in the late 1960s and early 1970s by Dr. Bernard Grad, in Canada, could (as did Olga Worrall) "heal" trypsin, an enzyme that breaks down protein when the trypsin had been extremely damaged mechanically. Dr. Grad also demonstrated remarkable healing by Mr. Esterbane of controlled-size skin wounds on rats.[8]

Mietek Wirkus, formerly of Poland and now living in Maryland near Washington D.C., has an outstanding reputation as a healer. Norm was able to obtain proof of his ability to heal individuals with severe hearing loss. Six patients showed impressive improvement in their audiograms after treatment with him. He prefers to work in tandem with physicians. Before emigrating from Poland, he worked primarily in Polish medical centers as a licensed bioenergy healer. He has been tested by Dr. Elmer Green of the Menninger Clinic; healing pulses sent by him have been measured at an astonishing eight volts. Wirkus has treated many prominent Washington residents, including members of congress.

Mietek Wirkus also participated in a controlled case study that used an EEG to measure the brain functions of a bioenergy practitioner and client during a healing experience, and also at a distance. The experimenters found that as areas of the practitioner's brain changed frequency, so did those of the subject, though the subject's frequencies were more variable than those of the practitioner. The practitioner's brain waves were more stable during distant healing, and less stable during present healing; they may have been affected by those of the client.[9] His web site is www.MietekWirkus.com.

Deena Spear is one of the more remarkable modern soul healers. A former neurobiologist, she coauthored several papers documenting the negative effects of pesticides on the environment. When she realized that laboratory chemicals were having an adverse effect on her own health, she began studying violin-making and acoustics. After two decades as a violin-maker, she discovered that she could change the sound and vibration of instruments mentally—without any tools. As she and her husband Robert Spear became well known in their craft, many of the professional musicians who played their instruments found they didn't have to travel to have their instruments adjusted; Deena discovered she could perform acoustical adjustments long distance. Dramatic changes in the power, quality, and playability of the musical instruments served as validation to both Deena and professional musicians (including world-renowned cellist Mstislav

Rostropovich, who bought a Spear cello) that she genuinely was able to telepathically enhance musical instrument sound. She found that she could apply the same skills with humans and animals to assist in their healing process. To Deena, whether a person's problems are physical or emotional, it's all a felt sound vibration.

She wrote *Ears of the Angels,* which humorously chronicles her journey from Cornell University-trained biologist, to professional violin maker, to professional healer. The book includes testimonials and histories of various healings, sometimes written by the clients themselves.[10]

For example, one of the first transplant cases she worked with showed a dramatic and lifesaving drop in the creatinine (a metabolic waste product) levels in the patient's blood after her long distance healing. Because of life-threatening infections, the patient's doctors had been forced to drastically reduce the amount of immunosuppressant drugs administered. The patient had received a kidney transplant seven years before, and had been taking immunosuppressants ever since, in order to stop her body from rejecting the transplanted kidney. Without her usual dose, the doctors expected the kidney to die and the level of blood waste products in her blood to soar.

After the healing, just the opposite occurred. The patient's physicians, who were not told about the healing, were quite puzzled by the turn of events. The kidney functioned better than ever, and her blood was cleaner—all at far lower dosages of immunosuppressant drugs than had been needed in the previous seven years.

Deena is also developing tools to help people shift consciousness. One involves a combination of music and language. EEG tests show that her recordings balance the right and left hemispheres of the brain. Christiane Northrup, M.D., writes this of Deena: "One of her students, Margaret Wells, M.D., specializes in occupational medicine, treating those who are injured on the job. Dr. Wells has been working most recently at workman's compensation clinics and has been using the healing skills she learned from Deena with tremendous success...

"During one week, six patients came to the emergency room at Dr. Wells' clinic with metal filings or other foreign bodies in their eyes. When metal filings enter the eye, they can leave a rust ring, which needs to be removed by scraping or drilling it out bit by bit.... Before attending Deena's workshops, Dr. Wells typically referred patients with this type of condition to an ophthalmologist. Since studying with Deena, she will tune her patient... Dr. Wells used vibrational healing to treat five of the six cases. She referred the sixth patient to an eye surgeon after sensing that he would not be receptive to the tuning. For the five men she treated, Dr. Wells reported that, 'The metal shards were removed easily. An exam the day after the procedures showed no visible abrasion or injury in the eyes of any of the five cases.' This is astounding because it generally takes several attempts to remove all the rust. And typically antibiotic drops are used through the night (often every hour), yet none of the people who received the tuning needed the eye drops or experienced any pain.

"Deena was quoted in an article for *Body & Soul* magazine saying, 'Almost everything in conventional medicine could be made better if energy healing were involved. The medicine of the future lies in understanding how we create health and illness—from thoughts and beliefs, which create the energy fields that create our bodies.' I couldn't agree more. And I also believe that in a century or two, people will look back at the kind of medicine practiced in our time and wonder why there was so little understanding—and use—of vibrational healing techniques."[11] Deena's web site is www.Singing-Woods.org.

Barbara Rasor, Ph.D., describes herself as an "emotional intuitive." She is good at getting to the root causes of a person's symptoms. A former MRI technician, she became a hypnotherapist, only to discover that she was intuitively picking up her clients' emotions and medical information. She began to develop her abilities, and research the science behind her perceptions. Barbara sees clients and also teaches at Holos University. Her web site is www. EmotionalIntuitive.com.

Cay Randall-May, Ph.D., does intuitive physical and energy body readings, followed by prayer, hands-on healing, or distant healing. She obtained a doctorate in Entomology from the University of California, Berkeley, before seeking ordination. Her postdoctoral research focused on the developmental interactions of nerve and muscle in arthropods, research that was equally valuable in understanding other animals and humans. She has taught at many institutions besides Berkeley; offering courses in anatomy and physiology, general biology, and scientific illustration.

As well as publishing dozens of scientific papers, articles, and essays, she has a book entitled *Pray Together Now: How to Find or Form a Prayer Group,* documenting her experiences with more than ninety prayer groups.[12] The groups were drawn from different faiths, as well as several Christian denominations. It lists many prayer resources and Internet sites.

The way she developed a belief in the healing power of prayer is interesting. She recounts these stories: "My family encouraged me, as a child, to say 'grace' before meals and prayers before I went to sleep. That's why it was natural for me, at about age twelve, to pray for my pet cat when he developed sores between the toes of his feet. The sores kept him from climbing the tree in my backyard where he and I spent lots of time together. As soon as I noticed he was in pain, I asked in my bedtime prayer for him to be restored to good health so he could play in the tree again. It didn't occur to me that such a request was far-fetched or unreasonable. The day after I prayed for him, he effortlessly scrambled up the tree. I looked closely at his paws and the sores were gone—overnight.

"Many years later, after I had gone through the University of California and obtained my graduate degrees in Entomology, I became ill and had to have surgery. The doctor warned me not to travel right away, but I was anxious to drive to my postdoctoral research position at Case Western Reserve University, in Cleveland, Ohio. Along the way I hemorrhaged—and found myself in hospital facing repeated surgery. This time I turned to prayer out of desperation. I imagined that I was focusing the healing energy of the universe into my body through prayer. After what seemed like hours of intense, solitary prayer, my inner mind was suddenly filled with the image of a huge hand wrapped around my midsection. At the same time I felt enormous heat fill my whole body. The internal bleeding stopped immediately. I was discharged, and resumed my car trip to Ohio without further incident."

During her sessions she holds a patient in a field of unconditional love. In her words, "I strive to reach a level of loving connection with the universal healing source and also with the individual requesting healing. It seems to me that the healing does not originate from within me, but passes through me like water through a pipeline." Her web site is www.PrayNow.net.

John Sewell is a remarkable spiritual healer who lives near Atlanta, Georgia. He has had great success with migraine headaches, PMS, and cancer. He believes that the more spiritual patients are initially, the faster they respond. He also believes that cancer is usually an effect; when he treats patients, he "asks the body" what caused it. "The body always wants to be well," he notices.

He lays people on a massage table, where he moves his hands over them; he can visually perceive energy drains. He then does muscle testing to confirm his observations. John believes that releasing trauma requires conscious awareness; otherwise his treatments are, "just a nice massage." So he endeavors to bring buried psychological traumas back to conscious memory. "Ninety-eight percent of ailments are emotionally based," he says. He needs to have patients present in person to read the emotions underlying the pain.

He also asks patients—via muscle testing—if they are ready to heal; he finds it often takes two or three sessions before enough trust is established to bring people to this point. If the trauma is just in a muscle, he finds it can release in two to 20 minutes.

Cancer tumors take longer; he finds that many dissolve in around four days. He has also discovered that if a patient has had a long course of chemotherapy, it is usually impossible to bring them back to health. He believes that spiritual healers need to work on patients before they have conventional cancer treatments, which he believes compromises their immune system, often beyond the point of no return. His experience is that cancer is usually caused by the person's attitude.

He has noticed that the body can clear up to three major emotional traumas in a session, at maximum. Then a week or more of rest and integration is required before tackling others. He has worked at spiritual healing hospitals in cities in Brazil, as well as spending two years with medicine men in the Amazon jungle. He noticed plenty of fakery in their methods, yet their patients got well anyway. He saw one medicine man use a goat's intestine in a supposed "psychic surgery." When he challenged the man, the shaman reminded John that the woman had recovered from her illness immediately afterward! The medicine man said, "Some people travel for two weeks to see me. Believing they will be healed, they start getting better on the way. When I touch them, it simply confirms the healing." There were hundreds of people in this village, all of them healthy—without the benefit of drugs other than native herbs, or surgery, other than the medicine man's theater.

John Sewell also muscle tests his clients for prescribed medications; he finds that while cholesterol-lowering drugs are often indicated, antidepressants are usually not. He also muscle tests them to determine if the supplements they are taking are desired by their bodies. He prefers to know nothing whatever about his clients. Sometimes, he says, "they walk in here with a thick file of medical records." He tells the person to set the file down, and get on the table; reassuring them that, "we'll compare notes later and see how good I am."

He does distant healing too, but he prefers to have patients present in person. He has found that distant healing addresses only the pain, and not the underlying emotions. When he does distant healing, he lies on his own table, and asks the patient to lie down at the same time. Again, he prefers no information other than the patient's address. He can tell their age and weight, hair color, and exactly where in their bodies the pain resides.

His gift began as a survival skill during a rough childhood. "I've always been able to stop bleeding, even as a little boy," he says. "When I was twelve years old, I was boating with some other kids my age. There were no adults around. My sister's ten-year-old friend fell while skiing, and the ski hit her in the thigh. She was thrashing around in pain, and we hauled her into the boat, crying and writhing. I stuck my fingers into the injured area. I felt a 'cloak' come over me, like a warm, light trance. The girl stopped crying and thrashing. Then I jumped in the water and yelled 'My turn!' I did it because I hadn't had a turn to ski yet! Later my sister said to me, 'Something got into you today, that's how you fixed her.'"

His survival skills got him through the Vietnam war; he afterwards decided that he would develop his healing gift with the intention of helping others. He chooses to keep himself in excellent shape in order to stay clear enough to do his work. He does not use alcohol, caffeine, sugar or salt. He also drinks lots of pure water and gets plenty of exercise. He avoids electromagnetic fields; he finds himself unable to work in hospitals, because of the high ambient levels of radiation, though he says, "nursing homes are okay."[13]

Unique though he may be, there are many aspects of John Sewell's practice and background that illuminate typical aspects of soul medicine. One of these is a childhood awareness of a healing gift. Another is a very strong intention to be of service. A third is a lifestyle that supports the maximization of his powers. A fourth is a focus on the underlying cause, and the perception of disease as a symptom. In the next chapter we will examine these and other characteristics of a master healer.

Donna Eden has done a great service to the field through her work, and through her best selling book *Energy Medicine*,[14] one of the most user-friendly and practical guides available in the field. She has mastered many different techniques of energy healing. She uses them with clients, and presents each of them clearly in her book. She is also exquisitely attuned to whether and where a person is ready for healing, yet she does not hesitate to prompt people in the direction of taking responsibility for their own wellness. Donna's passionate care for her clients and students shines through everything she does.

She tells the following story, which illuminates several aspects of her approach, about one of her first patients: "A woman with ovarian cancer came for a session with the hope that I could help relax her body and prepare it for a surgery that was scheduled in five days. She had been told to 'get her affairs in order' as her immune system was so weak that her chances of surviving the surgery were limited. Metastasis was also suspected.

"From looking at her energy, I was certain the cancer had not metastasized. While her energy was dim and collapsed close to her body, the only place that looked like cancer to me was in her left ovary. In addition, the texture and vibration and appearance of the energy coming up through her ovary was responsive to my work with her. I could see and feel it shift, and by the end of the session, the pain that had been with her for weeks was gone.

"I told her that her body was so responsive to what I had done that I wondered about her plan to have surgery. I was concerned that her immune system was indeed too weak, and I was confident that by working with her energy, not only would her immune system be strengthened, the tumor's growth could be reversed. While I made my statements with the strong disclaimers required to avoid immediate arrest for practicing medicine without a license, she responded to the implication that she cancel the surgery with horror. I suggested she at least delay the operation for two weeks. She scheduled a session with me for the next day and said she would discuss the surgery with her husband.

"That evening I received a call from her husband. He was outraged and threatening. He called me a 'quack.' He said I was putting his wife's life in jeopardy by giving her false hope, and he told me I would never have another chance to confuse her like this. He made it clear that she would not be coming back. When I began to respond, he hung up. I called back a short while later. She answered. Talking in hushed tones, she was clearly uncomfortable speaking with me. I said, 'Okay, don't postpone the surgery, but please keep your appointment tomorrow. You don't have to pay. You have nothing to lose. I believe in what I am saying. In fact, I want you to bring your husband in with you. Find a way!' She did not believe he would come in, but the next day, they both arrived for the appointment.

"I had her lie down on the massage table. My hope was to find a way to give this traditional and skeptical man, so poignantly fierce in his protection of his wife, an experience of healing energy that his senses could not deny. I could see a dark, dense energy at the site of his wife's left ovary, and it felt like my hand was moving through a muddy swamp. I asked the husband to place his hand a few inches above the area and begin to circle it, using a motion that tends to draw energy out of the body. To his great surprise, not only could he immediately feel that he was moving against something, within two minutes his hand was pulsing with pain. To his utter amazement, his wife reported that her pain diminished as his increased.

"By the end of the session she was again pain-free, felt better, and looked better. I had also been able to show them both, through the use of 'energy testing,' that we had been able to direct healing energies from her immune system to the area of her cancer. I taught him a set of procedures to use with her every day. They decided to temporarily postpone the surgery and ask for further medical tests prior to rescheduling it. After about ten days of these daily treatments from him and three more sessions with me, she went through the additional testing. The tumor was gone." Donna Eden and David Feinstein have a strong commitment to teaching others these methods, and they supplied the following story about the success of one of their students. With his permission, the patient's real name is used:

"Tim Garton, a world champion swimmer, was diagnosed in 1989 with Stage Two Non-Hodgkin's Lymphoma. He was forty-nine years old. He had a tumor the size of football in his abdomen. It was treated with surgery, followed by four chemotherapy treatments over twelve weeks, with subsequent abdominal radiation for eight weeks. Despite initial concern that the cancer appeared to be terminal, the treatment was successful, and by 1990, Time was told that he was in remission. He was also told that he would never again compete at a national or international level. However, in 1992, Tim Garton returned to competitive swimming, and won the one hundred meter freestyle world championship.

"In early July of 1999, he was diagnosed with prostate cancer. A prostatectomy in late July revealed that the cancer had expanded beyond the borders of his prostate and could not all be surgically removed. Once again, he received weekly radiation treatment in the area of his abdomen. After eight weeks of treatment, the cancer had cleared.

"In 2001, the lymphoma returned, this time in his neck. It was removed surgically. Tim again received radiation, though this time it left severe burns on his neck. The following year, a growth on the other side of his neck, moving over his trachea, was diagnosed as a fast-growing lymphoma that required emergency surgery.

"He was told that the lymphoma was widespread. A bone marrow and stem cell transplant, called an autogolus, was done at this time, but it was not successful. There was also concern that the tumors would metastacize to his stomach. His doctors determined at this point that they could do nothing more for him. He was told that highly experimental medical treatments, for which there was little optimism, were the only alternative. He was given an injection of monoclonal antibodies (Retuxin), which had been minimally approved for recurrent low-grade lymphoma. Retuxin is designed to flag the cancer sites and potentially help stimulate the immune system to know where to focus.

"At this point Tim enlisted the services of Kim Wedman, an energy medicine practitioner trained by Donna Eden. Tim and his wife went to the Bahamas for three weeks, and they brought Kim with them for the first week. Kim provided daily sessions

74

lasting an hour and a half. These sessions included a basic energy balancing routine, "meridian tracing," a "chakra clearing," work with the "electrical," "neurolymphatic," and "neurovascular" points, a correction for energies that are designed to cross over from one side of the body to the other but are not, and a daily assessment of his other basic energy systems, followed by corrections for any that were out of balance. While Tim was not willing to follow Kim's advice to curb his substantial alcohol consumption, or modify his meat-and-potatoes diet, he did introduce fresh vegetable juices into his regimen, plus a herbal tea (Flor-Essence) that is believed to have medicinal properties.

"Kim also taught Tim and his wife a twenty-minute, twice-daily energy medicine protocol, which they followed diligently, both during the week she was there, and for the subsequent two weeks. The protocol included a basic energy balancing routine, and specific interventions for the energy pathways that govern the immune system and that feed energy to the stomach, kidneys, and bladder.

"Upon returning to his home in Denver, in order to determine how quickly the cancers might be spreading, Tim scheduled a follow-up assessment with the oncologist who had told him, "There is nothing more that we can do for you." To everyone's thrill and surprise, Tim was cancer-free. He has remained so during the four years between that assessment and the time of this writing. He has been checked with a PT scan each year, with no cancer detected. Was it the energy treatments or the single Retuxin shot that caused the cancer to go into remission over those three weeks? No one knows. Tim still receives Retuxin injections every two months, but he also continues to work with Kim Wedman on occasion for tune-ups."

One of the more unusual healers that I (Norm Shealy) had an opportunity to meet and evaluate briefly is Reverend Bill Brown, originally a Presbyterian minister who became an "etheric surgeon." In the mid-1970s, I visited Brown in Georgia and observed his healing. He also treated my own neck problem.

Brown went into a very deep trance. Without actually touching my body, he went through motions as if injecting anesthesia, as well as various surgical maneuvers. His hands turned deep, almost beet red—and were extremely warm. Unfortunately I had no thermistors with me to measure the temperatures, which may have been well above his body temperature. Although Brown verbally reported many cures, I was never able to obtain medical records attesting to his ability to heal.

Several years ago I met Richard Gordon, who developed a technique that he calls *Quantum Touch*. The principles of Quantum Touch as outlined by Gordon are:

1. Energy follows thought. The practitioner uses intention and various meditations to raise and move the energy.

2. Breathing amplifies the life force.

3. The practitioner raises his or her vibration to create a high-energy field and uses that field to surround the area to be healed. Resonance and entrainment cause the area being healed to change vibration to match that of practitioner. The practitioner simply raises and holds the new resonance.

5. No one can really heal anyone else. The person in need of healing is the healer. The practitioner simply holds a resonance so that can happen.

6. The energy follows the body's intelligence to do the necessary healing. The practitioner pays attention to the body's intelligence and "chases the pain."

7. When energy moves through a blockage, it causes heat both in the practitioner and the patient.

8. The practitioner is also getting a healing by doing the work.

9. The ability to assist in healing is natural to all people.

10. Quantum Touch works well when combined with all other healing modalities.

11. Trust the process. The work may cause temporary pain or

other distressing symptoms that are all part of the healing. The life force and the healing process work with a complexity and wisdom that are beyond our conception.

When Richard Gordon visited us, he taught four people on our staff his technique, which consists of centering one's mind, detaching from all concerned, entering essentially a quiet meditative state, and beginning to feel one's own internal energy, *chi, qi,* or *prana,* moving from the legs up and out through the hands or fingers. Once one has this internal sensory process going, then the Quantum Touch therapist applies his or her hands near or around the areas where patients have difficulties. It may be to any part of the body from the top of the head to the tips of the toes. We also had Richard Gordon apply his Quantum Touch principles without touching the patient's body, and in three out of three situations he was clearly capable of altering the EEG during his sending of energy to the patient.

I have been fortunate to study and work with several remarkably talented intuitive diagnosticians, particularly Dr. Robert Leichtman and Dr. Caroline Myss. For more than a decade Caroline and I have been teaching a course in intuition. Increasingly, I receive requests for validation from people who claim to be medically intuitive; a few have great talent. Society is moving toward programs to train and authenticate those individuals who truly have medical intuitive capabilities; part of the purpose of this book is to spur such training and authentication.

I (Dawson Church) have had many provocative experiences with healers. Overcoming my skepticism has been a challenge for me, because while every "healer" seems to have plenty of dramatic anecdotes, there are rarely medically objective proofs of the patient's recovery; hence the focus on verifiable medical records in this book.

One exception is Peter Selby. Peter is a former physical therapist. Peter, and his wife Anne, travel widely, teaching and offering healing sessions. What makes their work unique is that changes to a client's body can be precisely measured immediately after a session, and Peter and Anne do just this.

Peter has a massage table set up in the front of the room during his demonstrations. When a person steps forward for healing, he measures the degree of rotation of various joints in their bodies. For instance, he might have the person raise their arms, and see how far back each arm rotates. He might have them sit on the table and look to the left, and measure how far their head rotates to the left, for instance, about 45 degrees. He usually picks a joint that is particularly constrained.

He and Anne then stand about ten feet from the client, and appear to go into a light trance while they work on connecting the person up to their soul source, and removing blockages to the free flow of energy.

After treatment is complete, they then measure the rotation of the same joints, to see if there is a difference. I watched them work on about twenty people, and there was always significantly greater mobility after the treatment. One woman had been in an auto accident many years before, and could only turn her head about 15 degrees to the right, and about 30 degrees to the left. She was most skeptical, and expressed little hope that she could be helped by them; after all, she said, "The injury is so old, and my body's used to it!" After treatment, she could turn her head about 45 degrees to both right and left, to her amazement.

I lay on the table and they measured the degree of rotation of my hip joints—a portion of my anatomy to which I had never before given a moment's thought. I raised my right leg, bent my knee, placed my right foot on my left knee, and rotated my right femur as far as possible. It rotated out to about 60 degrees. Well and good.

Then I reversed positions, and tested my left leg. It could only rotate about 30 degrees. I was dismayed that I did not have more flexibility—and that I did not even realize I did not have such flexibility. Then Peter and Anne stepped back about ten feet, and did a twenty minute treatment, focusing on my rigid left side, after which I climbed back on the table. My right leg could now rotate out 90 degrees, a significant improvement. But my left leg simply dropped to all the way to the table. "Good," observed Peter, "That one's horizontal too now."

"Wait," I responded, "I can feel that this is not the limit of travel. It can go further." I scooted till my left leg was hanging over the side of the table. It dropped still further, coming to rest at about 110 degrees. Two years later, both legs still have the same degree of rotation; the healing was permanent.

While the Selby's use joint rotation to test the effectiveness of their treatments, and while I would not hesitate to recommend treatment by them of anyone who has joint problems, their focus is not on producing more flexible bodies. It is instead on resolving the core emotional and spiritual wounds that are keeping the body locked up. They work directly on those issues, not on the joints themselves. Joint testing is simply a graphic demonstration that the client's energy has shifted. Details of the Selby's methods, and their contact information, can be found on their web site, www.YouAngelYou. com.

Psychic Surgeons

"Psychic surgery" is done primarily in the Philippines and Brazil. In September 1976, I (Norm Shealy) was a participant in a team (with Elmer Green of the Menninger Clinic, another physician, and a film crew) that visited seven psychic surgeons in the Philippines who perform surgery without tools other than their minds and hands. Six of the healers produced what appeared to be blood on the surface of the skin of their patients during the psychic surgery. I was able to take those blood samples from twenty-two of the patients by swabbing with cotton. All the samples proved later to be human blood.

I saw three specific types of psychic surgeons. Two individuals went into deep trances. Their eyes rolled up into their heads and fluttered as they worked. More commonly the healer did not seem to go into a trance and could carry on a perfectly normal conversation with us during the healing process.

One of these psychic surgeons, Tony Santiago, treated a male patient whose bladder cancer was significant enough to be seen through his thin skin. As Santiago placed his hands on the patient's abdomen, liquid blood and blood clots about the size of small popcorn popped out and splattered all over the room. I was able to collect a number of these clots, and they indeed were human blood. However, the size of the tumor did not change visibly.

There were two cameras focused on Santiago and three scientific observers watching. It was quite clear there was no sleight of hand. Santiago's pulse escalated to about 135 beats per second at the height of his healing.

Tony Agpaou, at that time the best-known healer in the Philippines, said to me, "You know, Norman, we only do these materializations because they give the patients faith in our ability." With that, he moved his hands about a foot apart and held them over the abdomen of a woman who did not speak English. As I looked down, it seemed as if her abdomen were opening, revealing the peritoneum, a shiny transparent membrane inside the abdomen that covers the organs. I could even see what looked like omentum, a fatty layer, through the peritoneum. I got down on my knees. The image I was seeing was at least a centimeter above her abdomen, not even touching it. Without moving his hands, Agpaou said, "And, just as we can materialize, we can dematerialize." The image then disappeared.

On a number of occasions over the course of an entire day, Agpaou materialized not only liquid blood but sometimes blood clots and at times bits of white tissue that looked like fascia, which is the substance between tissue planes within the body. He had on a short-sleeved shirt that could not hide anything. I followed him around, even going into the bathroom with him. I was allowed to look under the top of the table and in drawers in the room where he worked. He probably "produced" three pints of blood from various patients treated during that day.

One of the most interesting healers in the Philippines, known as Padre Tierte, worked in a small sanctuary where we witnessed him removing blood. He also removed some foul-smelling material, more than a pint in volume, from a woman's back. Smelling like the worst kind of rotting marsh, it is hard to believe something like that could have been hidden in the room. The aroma was so strong that I almost vomited when it appeared.

A fascinating event occurred when another psychic surgeon, named Jun Labou, worked on Alan Neuman, the producer of the television program that was being recorded during our trip. Labou told Neuman that he had mucus on his heart. Working primarily on Neuman's neck, Labou placed his hands deep between the trachea and the sternocleidomastoid muscle. Out poured at least several ounces of pure pus. He massaged the skin over the upper chest and more pus came out of Neuman, then at the end a few drops of blood. It looked very much as if an abscess had been opened by a surgeon's knife. I obtained samples of this, and it proved to be pus with many white blood cells present. I do not know any way in which pus can be stored and produced on call, with a few drops of blood then appearing, as happens when an abscess under pressure is opened. It is difficult to be certain that any healing took place as there was no medical evaluation earlier.

A year after our visit to the Philippines, Jun Labou was brought to our clinic (at that time in LaCrosse, Wisconsin), where he performed psychic surgical procedures on seventeen patients. Again, blood appeared. I was able to obtain samples of blood from two of the patients, as well as the blood that Labou removed. Also, I obtained a sample of Labou's blood. A forensic pathologist in Berkeley, California, who examined the samples, assured me that in each case the blood was that particular patient's blood type and not Jun Labou's blood.

During these procedures, I never personally saw a patient's skin actually open. It was always as if the blood were welling up, as if it were coming through the skin. Some Brazilian and Philippine films of psychic surgery do show possible openings of the skin; however, no scar or evidence of the procedure is visible on the patient's skin at the conclusion of the procedure.

81

Here is the story of a most unusual shaman, Daniel, who works physically and spiritually to accomplish remarkable healing experience, as told by a friend who has given us permission to share her story.

A Healing Journey: Tulum, December, 2005

The Beginning: I picked up the phone when it rang and heard a familiar voice on the other end, "We're planning a trip in December to Tulum in the Yucatan, to work with Daniel, the Mayan Shaman. I thought of your foot. Would you like to go with us?" I started to give her my standard answer, "I don't *do* Shamans," but the words would not come out of my mouth. Instead from within came a clear command, "Go!" It was so strong that I found myself immediately agreeing to go.

The Background: At the end of December, 2004, I had undergone serious re-construction of my left foot. The tendon that holds the ankle upright and provides an arch to the foot was basically gone. The surgeon was highly skilled and the surgery went well. By all accounts it was a "perfect" job. I ended up with a triple bone fusion in the foot and two large screws in the ankle. However, a year later I was still experiencing considerable pain in that foot, and also in my right hip (I assume due to compensations made for the foot pain). I continued to participate in a number of therapies: chiropractic, massage, Rolfing, visualization and exercise. This kept me mobile—but the foot still felt as if it didn't belong to me. Putting weight on it was very painful. I went down stairs sideways, and I needed the constant support of a shoe.

The Journey: Most of those who call themselves "Shamans" work within the prescribed cultural patterns of their own traditional beliefs. A person coming from "outside" that tradition or belief may or may not resonate with the experience. The ability to traverse multiple levels of reality is part of this tradition. How those levels of reality are experienced and described depends, in large part, on one's cultural traditions. I had no idea how a Mayan shaman would approach his work, but somehow I had a deep inner knowing that whatever happened was the next step for me at this point in time.

The Place: Tulum is on the Caribbean shore near Cancun, Mexico, with white sands and aqua sea. The cabanas where we stayed were comfortable, but modest. There was no electricity in the cabanas, so it was candlelight (or flashlight) after dark. This created a very restful atmosphere and a re-establishment of natural rhythms (We generally went to bed at dark and woke up at dawn). The sea breezes and the sound of ocean waves graced our cabana.

The Work: I experienced five one-hour sessions with Daniel. These sessions are not easy to describe since so much was happening on so many levels. On the purely physical level, Daniel's approach might be described as *the most* intense Rolfing and deep tissue work I have ever experienced. It soon became clear that he had no intention of backing off until every part of my foot that was still meant to move, moved. He worked over my right hip in the same way. He did intense work on my spinal alignment. In addition, he offered energy work and heart-felt prayers. There were times when I felt that if the deep tissue work went any deeper I would simply let out a blood-curdling scream. At the same time I sensed his uncanny ability to "see inside" and really know the territory in which he was working. So, I did my best to "breathe through it".

He noticed on the first day that, when I lay on my stomach, I dropped my left foot off the side of the table (I could not flex it enough to lay it flat on its face). So that's where he started. By the end of the session my foot was lying very flat, face down, totally relaxed. He was delighted. I couldn't believe I had lived through it. I noticed his personal energy felt similar to that of other genuine healers with whom I have worked and that he occasionally had me take three breaths.

On each of the days there was a change in my body for the better. He worked the whole body but concentrated on the left foot and right hip. On the third day, I awakened with my two feet cradled together. My left foot felt like a part of me for the first time since the surgery! I awakened laughing, after a wonderful dream.

After my last session with this sincere and humble healer, I surprised myself by bursting into tears when I tried to say goodbye. He gave me a warm hug and said, in Spanish, "Don't be sad. I am your brother and you are my sister and there can never be any distance between us."

A Month Later: What Daniel was able to accomplish has remained: tremendously more flexibility in my foot, and no pain in my hip. If I am on my foot working for seven or eight hours, it becomes a bit painful in the uppercenter. My gait feels natural now, and my foot feels like *my* foot. That is the greatest change. Somehow, increasing the flexibility in all the joints and ligaments that still move took a lot of pressure off the front joint.

Daniel told our group that, a number of years previously, he was in a near-fatal accident. He suffered broken bones, many torn ligaments, and other injuries. During his recovery, he had a near-death experience. He describes it this way: "I found myself in the stars with my Master. I pleaded to be able to stay in the stars with him, but he told me I had to return to do special work. He showed me the healing I would do through his Spirit. When I became conscious, I refused to be taken to a hospital. I was taken home and healed through guidance from my Master's Spirit. I was told exactly what to do to heal the broken ribs and other injuries. After that, I began my work with other people. I do not know what name you would give the one who is my Master. To me he is Jesus Christ." Daniel works outside of any religious rationale or cultural story. As with all true healers, he simply allows Spirit to work through him.

Daniel's own Mayan culture doesn't understand what he does, though the surrounding Mayans come to him for healing. During a special ceremony with our group, he said that this was the first time since his experience *en las estrellas* (in the stars) with his Master that he had actually been able to share his story fully and honestly with a group of people. He told us, with gratitude, "Now I no longer feel like an orphan." The story of his life demonstrates our potential for healing, transformation, and transcendence through the power of love.

The Importance of Attitude

Rod Campbell, a healer from New Zealand, has worked on a number of patients at our clinic on several occasions. He says, "The people who have permanent recoveries, even after being told there was nothing medical science could do for them, are the people who have a complete change of attitude. After being told they have a very short time to live, they then see and appreciate the little things they never had time to see before."[16]

Although Edgar Cayce was not a healer in the usual sense, he did almost 10,000 trance readings related to health and illness. Scores of books have been written about his work. Cayce emphasizes that all healing ultimately is spiritual, involving atonement with God or a divine force, assisted by the patient's attitude, by physicians of various persuasions, or by prayer or sacred healers. His most frequent spiritual message was:

- Know that all strength, all healing of every nature is the changing of the vibrations from within-the attuning of the Divine within the living tissue of a body to Creative Energies. This alone is healing. Whether it is accomplished by the use of drugs, the knife, or whatnot, it is the attuning of the atomic structure of the living cellular force to its spiritual heritage.[17]

Some other observations from his readings also give us clues about what's happening in the course of soul medicine:

- But if your mind holds to it, and you've got a stumped toe, it will stay stumped. If you've got a bad condition in your gizzard, or liver, you'll keep it if you think so.[18]

- Medications only attune or accord a body for the proper reactions from the elemental forces of divinity within each corpuscle, each cell, each activity of every atom of the body itself.[19]

- No mechanical appliance does the healing. It only attunes

the body to a perfect coordination and the Divine gives the healing. For life is divine, and each atom in a body that becomes cut off by disease, distrust or an injury, then only needs awakening to its necessity of coordination, cooperation with the other portions that are divine, to fulfill the purpose which the body, the soul, came into being.[20]

- Thus does spiritual or psychic influence of body upon body bring healing to any individual; when another body may raise that necessary influence in the hormone of the circulatory forces as to take from that within itself to revivify or resuscitate diseased, disordered or distressed conditions within a body.[21]

On the web site of the American Board of Scientific Medical Intuition, you can find a list of those who have passed the national board certification exam as Counseling Intuitives: www.absmi.com.

Verifiable Medical Documentation

One of Ostad Parvarandeh's great contributions to the study of soul medicine is that so many of his cures were supported by medical documentation. In addition to the case history summaries we have already provided, medical records confirm that Ostad also healed patients with:

- osteogenic sarcoma, the most malignant form of cancer, not curable with any chemotherapy;
- neuroblastoma in a six-month-old child;
- adenocarcinoma of the stomach in a sixty-six-year-old man (stomach cancer is rarely cured with surgery or chemotherapy);
- spinal cord tumor not curable medically;
- hepatitis within ten days, with liver enzymes returning to normal;

- a ruptured intervertebral disc for which only surgery had been recommended;

- Forty percent recovery of visual fields in a man who originally was approximately 90 percent blind from retinitis pigmentosa;

- severe glaucoma (cured from a long distance);

- Hepatitis B;

- Gilles de la Tourette's syndrome;

- breast cancer metastatic to bone, in a thirty-eight-year-old woman;

- a spinal cord tumor diagnosed by MRI (magnetic resonance imaging), along with perhaps a slight residual scar, in a forty-six-year-old man diagnosed by a leading American neurosurgeon, and

- A cystic lesion of the pineal; the woman's cyst disappeared completely.

Divine energy travels instantly through time and space and can be directed by such talented individuals, whatever their faith and beliefs might be. James Oschman reports on studies of healers from many different traditions, including a Christain faith healer, a Hawaiian kahuna, ESP readers, and seers: "In 1969, Robert C. Beck began a decade of research on the brain wave activity of 'healers' from a wide variety of subcultures... [recording] their electrical brain waves with an EEG. All the healers produced similar brain wave patterns when they were in the 'altered state' and performed a 'healing'... [they] produced nearly identical EEG signatures..."[22] It appears that master healers everywhere are able to gain access to a level of soul consciousness that opens the doors to healing. Pioneering psychiatrist Stanislav Grof recently wrote, "It is hard to imagine that Western academic science will continue indefinitely to censor all the extraordinary evidence that has in the past been accumulated...as well as to ignore the influx of new data." As the trickle of data becomes a flood, science is beginning to map the processes at work when master healers work their apparent magic.

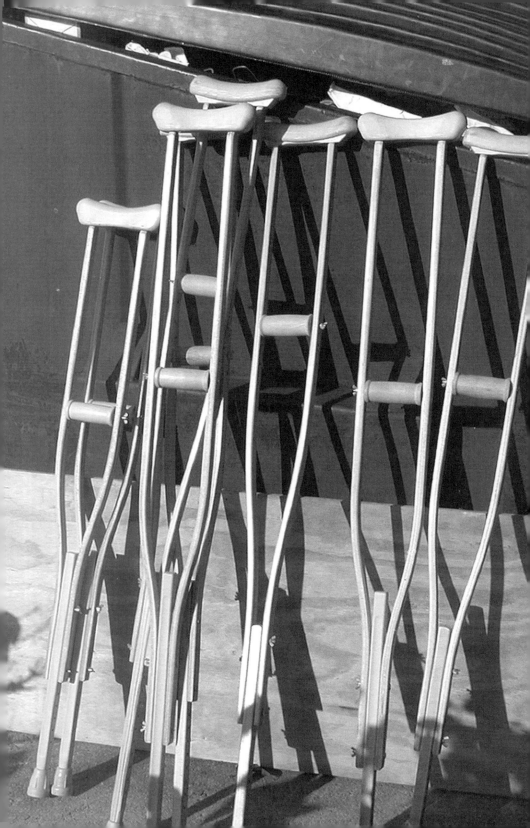

6

Characteristics of a Master Healer

Why can a healer's presence effect healing, while the presence of another person cannot? There are a number of characteristics that emerge, both from scientific studies of healers and healing, and also from their own writings and teachings. While the effectiveness of healers may vary greatly, there are definable characteristics common to master healers.

Most healers do not see themselves as special. They emphasize that everyone has these abilities, even though they may have cultivated them to a heightened degree. By studying them, we can learn a great deal about the elements common to all great healers, as well as cultivating a healing presence in our daily lives.

Calm Emotional States

Our hearts do not beat in a regular rhythm. Heart rate varies continually, slowing up and speeding down. The degree of fluctuation, measured on an electrocardiogram, is called *heart rate variability*. The degree of heart rate variability we experience at any given moment correlates closely with our emotional state. Anger, fear, anxiety and frustration are associated with a disordered heart rhythm, a high degree of heart rate variability. Emotional states such as love, peace, compassion and tranquility are associated with decreases in heart rate variability, and a more stable, consistent rhythm.[1]

Healers typically have a strong spiritual practice and belief system. Those who regularly induce feelings of peace and tranquility in themselves—and have a spiritual practice focusing on love and compassion—are more likely to enter the kind of physiological state associated with healing. On a physical level, a master healer is likely to be adept at entering this state of "heart coherence." Buddhist meditation emphasizes tranquility as an essential prerequisite to connecting our minds and hearts with the all that is. A master healer, in the healing state, is typically tranquil inside, even if their outer actions are animated. Even though aspects of their daily lives—marriages, money, children—may be as messy as the average person, when they enter the healing space, they shift to a place of inner serenity.

Intention

The experimenters at the Hearthmath Institute who studied the effect of consciousness on DNA found that, in order to affect its molecular angles, a subject required more than a state of heart congruence. It also required *intention*. Heart congruence without intention did not effect a change in DNA. Intention without heart congruence was equally ineffective. But intention projected from a tranquil, compassionate state was effective indeed.

As well as entering a tranquil internal state, the master healer needs to have a strong and clear intention to heal. John of God, João Teixeira da Faria, is a famous faith healer in Brazil. Though his healing is done while he is in a trance, and unaware of what is occurring around him, he uses many traditional Catholic formulations and concepts in his mission. There are thousands of testimonials of people cured of all kinds of diseases after visiting him—stage four terminal cancer, depression, herniated disks, multiple sclerosis, brain tumors, gallstones, cataracts, chronic arthritis, leukemia, and cardiovascular failure. In one room of his compound, there is a ceiling-high stack of crutches, wheelchairs and braces paying silent testimony to his success.[2] Fans include Shirley MacLaine and several sports stars who have been cured from sports-related injuries. ABC news, one of the "Big Four" US news organizations, followed the cases of several people who went to see John of God. Here's how they reported their findings:

"Matthew Ireland, of Guilford, Vermont, was told he had a quick-growing inoperable brain tumor. He had undergone radiation and chemotherapy treatments. But almost two years after he was diagnosed, and after three visits with João, his tumor has shrunk.

"Annabel Sclippa of Boulder, Colorado, has not been able to walk since her spinal cord was nearly severed in a car crash in 1988. But after six visits with João, she says she can now feel sensation in her legs and can nearly balance herself standing between handrails—something her physiotherapist said was unusual with her type of injury.

"Mary Hendrickson of Seattle was diagnosed with chronic fatigue syndrome and powerfully debilitating allergies. She now feels much more energetic. 'There is no way I would feel this way if something hadn't changed inside me,' she told 'Primetime Live.' 'Something's made a difference.'

"David Ames, of San Francisco, was diagnosed with Lou Gehrig's disease in April 2003. His nervous system was slowly disintegrating, and he faced almost certain death—only 10 percent of patients survive for 10 years or more. He has had no physical improvement, but he still says his spirit has gained from his visit.

"Lisa Melman of Johannesburg, South Africa, discovered a year ago that she had breast cancer. After visiting João, her doctor told her it had grown, although less aggressively than he expected it to and that she should still have surgery."[3]

Thousands of pilgrims flock to the town of Abadiania where Joao practices. Sometimes it is almost impossible to get into his compound, the *casa,* or to obtain individual attention. So he occasionally practices mass healings.[4] There are reports of him walking into a room containing over a hundred people, and declaring, "In the name of the Father, Son, and Holy Spirit, you are healed." His intention is big enough to encompass a roomful of people.

In his book *The Secret Life of Plants,* Christopher Bird was one of the first writers to provide dramatic scientific evidence of the power of intention. He describes experiments in which a rubber plant was hooked up to a polygraph. The researchers wanted to see if they could obtain a reading by cutting the plant's leaves. They discovered that they could not. They were startled, however, when they happened to glance further back at the polygraph recording, and discover that the plant had registered a large reaction when they *thought* of cutting its leaves.[5]

Healers often move into intense states of concentration while performing their work. The act of entering a still, prayerful state sets the ground for intention. Intention then becomes the vehicle through which the power of healing can move. Visualization, imagining, "outpicturing," and having a mental equivalent of the physical change you would like to see; any of these may occur in a state of intention. There may be a correlation between the strength of intention and the size of the effect, though our abilities to study such a possibility scientifically are still a long way off.

Master healers may have the ability to project extremely strong intentions. Most people, on the other hand, do not have a great deal of power behind their intentions. New Year's resolutions famously fall flat. Feeble prayers for peace are often undone by the fierce rush to war. If wishes were horses, beggars would ride.

If most intentions produce no result, how can the intentions of master healers be so effective?

In the Evangelical Christian tradition, master healers are called "faith healers." This term recognizes the crucial role that faith and belief plays in healing. Desmond Tutu, Archbishop of Cape Town, and a man who by faith alone was able to play a pivotal role in the healing and emancipation of the entire country of South Africa, said, "There is more to be done, some days, than I can possibly accomplish. On such mornings I realize I must then spend an extra hour in prayer." Tutu looked to God, when there was no possibility that human solutions could unravel the knot of hatred, repression, and political violence in which his country was entangled. Faith can move governments, and it can certainly move bodies; as Jesus said, "Thy faith hath made thee whole."

Healers may hold an intention for a sick person even when that person is incapable of holding that intention themselves. Believing in the possibility of healing, even when all evidence points to the contrary, may eventually swing all the healing systems of body, mind and soul into alignment with the intention. One study, also performed by the Heartmath Institute, examined the production of Immunoglobulin-A. This is an immune factor easily studied through its concentration in the saliva. Immunoglobulin-A is "the body's first line of defense against viruses and bacteria in the lungs, digestive and urinary tracts."[6]

Subjects in the study spent just five minutes each morning harboring positive thoughts. Their levels of Immunoglobulin-A spiked upward sharply, indicating increased immune system response. The surprising fact, however, was that the effect of that one brief period lasted throughout the day. Levels dropped slowly; by the afternoon, they still had elevated levels of immune factors in their systems.[7]

The subjects were instructed to pick a thought that triggered positive emotions in them. It did not matter whether the subjects were triggered thinking about the Buddha, their favorite pet hamster, Amnesty International, Tinkerbell, Jesus, their kind grandmother, Jesse Jackson, Allah, Wakantanka, a ski trip to Lake Tahoe, Ramakrishna, or their fairy Godmother. It's not *which* faith we hold that's important; it's *that* we hold faith that's important.

The flip side of the coin is that subjects who remembered an angry feeling, and replayed it in their minds for even five minutes, had a decreased production of Immunoglobulin-A. And the immune system suppression didn't just last during the brief period in which they remembered the anger. It significantly depressed the functioning of their immune system for the rest of that day. Hearthmath research director Rollin McCraty, one of the authors of the study, says, "This shows just how powerful self-induced emotions are, and could explain why colds and flu spread so fast through a stressful office. Reliving negative emotions depletes the power of the immune system for hours and hours, while reliving positive emotions boosts immune strength."[8]

Healers may "keep the faith" for sick people who have abandoned hope, and given up the attempt to hold a picture of a positive outcome for themselves. Victor Krivorotov, a Russian faith-healer-turned-psychologist, after examining hundreds of cases of faith healing, and participating in several scientific studies, declared that by entering the presence of a master healer, the energy systems of a patient could be reorganized, as they "borrowed faith" from a person with a strong healing intention.[9] In a chapter called "Love Therapy," he says that, "The most effective method of treatment involves a resonance between patient and healer, such that the malfunctioning subsystem, or all subsystems of the patient, begin to function in unison with the corresponding subsystems of the healer, which leads to a cure. The high spiritual potential of the healer can instantly bring all of the patient's subsystems into a harmonious state."

The marriage of intention and heart congruence has a powerful healing effect. Healing may be intention projected into the body.

Spiritual Practice

Most master healers are rooted in their faith tradition. Whether they are a Christian, Muslim Buddhist, Hindu or Jew, the religion they practice has less significance than their practice of religion.

Yet a master healer is unlikely to be an occasional or superficial practitioner; he or she is likely to be a passionate lover of God. Master healers aren't simply people who observe the dead formalities of their church; instead, the living stream of their faith tradition flows through them. They are people at the vibrant center of their religions, as well as having spirit at the center of their lives. Their spirituality is not something they do; their spirituality is who they are.

One of the keys to such spiritual vibrancy is *consistency*. Meditating once in a while can bring great peace, but daily meditation brings great power. Going back to the divine, over and over again, indicates that the divine is the source of one's answers and actions. A master healer's life of prayer and devotion produces a strong connection with divine energy. While many of us have flashes of spiritual enlightenment, moments when we enter a peak state, a master healer sets up his or her life to practice such attunement consistently. It means turning prayer into a lifestyle, rather than an occasional recourse. Master Sha is blunt about this. He says, "A lower-level soul does not have the coin of the realm in the Soul World and cannot get the attention of a high-level saint. This coin of the realm is virtue accumulated through service. A low-level soul has not performed enough service for others, has not given enough or helped enough or cared enough. However...a person who has performed service, prayer, and acts of kindness and goodness for others will have accumulated much greater merit. ...the saints will pay attention."[10]

Ostad Parvarandeh, a Muslim, taught that a true healer had to live a life of sacred behavior. To him, that meant abstaining from smoking, alcohol, or sexual excess. It also meant abstaining from anger. Turning to God when we're in crisis can give us a connection to a source of divine reality in which healing is possible. It opens a channel that is a small fraction of our total consciousness. When we go to God every day, we widen the channel; eventually it consumes our consciousness in the ecstasy of continual connection. Master healers, in this way, have reliable access to dimensions of reality that unpracticed spiritual seekers can barely touch. Consistency of spiritual practice is essential; far more important than the variety of religion through which you facilitate a contact with the divine."[11]

Distant Effects

A master healer need not be present in the room or even in the vicinity of a patient in order to have an effect. Ostad healed patients residing in London, England, while he was in San Francisco, California. Healing from a distance occurs instantaneously, completely outside our usual conceptual parameters of time and space. Time and distance play no part in a master healer's effect on a patient.

Some master healers can diagnose what is wrong with an individual by hearing the patient's voice on a tape or over a telephone, by seeing a photograph, preferably of the entire front and back of the body, or by knowing the full name of the individual. A diagnosis will include all known diseases, but sometimes will give information about a disease that has not yet become diagnosable by conventional means.

Some master healers use surrogates for distant healing. The surrogate assumes the role of the person being healed. The healer works on the surrogate as though that person were the subject, and the subject then experiences the effects of the master healer's work. Richard Geggie, a cardiac patient, relates the following extraordinary experience of distant healing by Pomo Indian healer, Lorin Smith:

"In the early 1990s I was in Toronto, Canada. I went to see my doctor because I felt tired and listless. He sent me to have an electrocardiogram. Later that day, when he got the results back, he told me that my heart was at serious risk. He told me to stay calm, not exert myself, keep nitroglycerine pills with me at all times, and to not go outside alone.

"The doctors administered several tests over the course of the following three days, and I failed them all because my arteries were severely clogged. They included a fluoroscope examination, another electrocardiagram, and a treadmill stress test. When I started the bicycle test, the clinic staff didn't even let me finish. They stopped me part way. They were afraid I was going to die on the spot, my arteries were so clogged. As a high risk patient, I was given an immediate appointment for heart bypass surgery.

"The day before the surgery, I woke up feeling much better. I went to the hospital and I was given an angiogram. This involved shooting dye into my arteries through an injection in my thigh. The surgeons wanted to discover the exact location of the blockages prior to the operation. I was prepared for surgery. My chest was shaved, and the doctors were about to mark my skin where they planned to make the incision. When the new angiograms came back from the lab, the doctor in charge looked at them. He became very upset. He said he had wasted his time. There were no blockages visible at all. He said he wished his own arteries looked as clear. He could not explain why all the other tests had shown such severe problems.

"I later discovered that my friend Lorin Smith in California, upon hearing of my heart trouble, had assembled a group of his students for a healing ceremony the day before the second angiogram. He covered one man with bay leaves and told him that his name was Richard Geggie. For the next hour, Lorin led the group in songs, prayers and movement. The next day, I was healed.

"I have seen Lorin facilitate other amazing healings. Sometimes he works in a trance, invoking his grandfather, Tom Smith, who was a very famous healer. When he emerges from trance, he's unable to remember what he has said."

Richard Geggie recounted this story some thirteen years later, for the book *The Heart of Healing*, still in excellent health.[12]

When in a state of tranquility, holding a strong intention, and projecting the power of a consistent spiritual practice, a master healer enters the state of quantum reality. Quantum reality is not bound by the perceptions of time and space that limit our experience in a Newtonian universe. Healing simply *is,* and time and space conform to the present moment *is*-ness of the quantum universe. According to Ostad, Einstein's famous equation, $e=mc^2$ (Energy = mass, times a constant squared), is perfectly reflected in the healing process. He postulated that spiritual healing converts mass into energy. The dissolution of a cyst or tumor is an example of mass—the diseased tissues—being converted into energy. The creation of new cells, such as the cure of cirrhosis of the liver, is an example of energy being converted into mass. These effects are not dependant on physical or temporal proximity of the healer. Dr. Zhi Gang Sha, though a remarkable healer and spiritual teacher, studied under a traditional Chinese doctor, Dr. Guo, in addition to getting a conventional Western medical degree. He says, "Dr. Guo has combined fifty years of clinical research with his own remarkable medical intuitive faculties in discovering a vital transfer mechanism between matter and energy at the cellular level. A quantum discovery, this transfer mechanism uses the space available in the body, the gaps between cells and between organs, to keep the body and its energy flow healthy."[13]

Transferability

Some healers can transfer their healing power to others. In a number of cases, Ostad Paravandeh came to trust a particular individual associated with a patient, such as a daughter caring for a parent. He was able to convey his ability to that individual, even across distances. The representatives are then deputized to perform certain healing techniques or the healing of specific diseases. The healer seems to have the power to grant permission to others to tap into his or her energy bank.

With the healer's permission, students or others are able to work with the energy systems of other individuals. Master Zhi Gang Sha will often "download" to a student the ability to convey healing to a loved one. Such deputized individuals seem to carry healing powers similar to those of the master.

Individuation

A master healer does not catch the patient's illness during the healing session. Furthermore, the healer does not have to muster his or her own energy to heal. An authentic healer never loses energy and is never fatigued or de-energized during the process. Master Zhi Gang Sha's students are amazed that even after fifteen to eighteen hours, he is still going strong, and will have the same degree of energy the following day and week, year after year. But he does not get involved with his patients. He does not even permit them to hug him. He has a strong sense of himself, and a firmly established sense of self as separate and apart from his patients. This ability to *individuate*—to separate oneself from entanglement with the morass of need and temptation that swirls around a master healer—is essential to maintaining these abilities.

The Emissary healing tradition of "attunement" has the healer call in the spirit of God, a master, or of a particularly beloved saint, to perform the healing. Jesus, or Maitreya, or Kwan Yin or St. Jude is invited to be present in the room. Rather than drawing on the limited conscious understanding of that particular human mind, the infinite capacities of the master are invoked. The master also deals with any dark energies that are present in the patient, energies that might overwhelm the capacities of the novice healer. There are accounts of healing that Jesus was able to perform in cases where his disciples were ineffective. The Gospel writer Matthew recounts a story of a man whose son had seizures. His distraught father came to Jesus and told him that his son had fallen into fire and into water, and suffered greatly. He plaintively tells the master: "And I brought him to your disciples, but they could not cure him." Matthew goes on to tell us that Jesus "rebuked the demon, devil, and he departed out" of the boy, who "was cured from that very hour."[14] Jesus was able to separate the disease out of the boy, without taking it on himself.

Master healers always refer back to their divine source, rather than claiming credit for healing. This may look like modesty or humility in the healer; in reality it creates the divine connection that is essential in maintaining healing power over time. Jesus, who must rank as one of the great healers of all time quite apart from his religious significance, said, "the Father that dwelleth in me, he doeth the works."[15]

Healers who are not master healers may take on some aspect of the patient's disease, and may eventually burn out or get sick. There are many accounts of healers who ran out of magic. When a healer becomes famous, and large amounts of money and adoration come his way, it is easy for a healer to begin thinking that he is special, and for his ego to swell to the point where it obscures his view of God.

Aimee Semple McPherson was one of the biggest faith healers of the 1920s. Her Foursquare Gospel Church in Los Angeles seated 5,000 people. She kept a museum of wheelchairs and crutches as evidence of her powers. However, she eventually had an affair with an associate, Kenneth Ormiston. She ran away with him for a month, and then covered it up with a story about having been kidnapped. She fell out of favor with press and congregants, and was found dead of an overdose of barbiturates in 1944. She failed the ultimate requirement of being a master healer.

Chogyam Trungpa, a Buddhist teacher who set popular culture aflame with his best seller *The Myth of Freedom,* was eventually exposed as an alcoholic and womanizer. He chose, as a successor to lead his order, a disciple who proceeded to sleep with many of his students, infecting several with AIDS.

McPherson and Trungpa are troubling examples, but they are not alone. The history of every religion is littered with biographies of healers and spiritual adepts who lost their way. Michael Peter Langevin has been the owner and editor of *Magical Blend* magazine for over a quarter-century. In that capacity, he has seen many sensational healers come and go. He writes:

"Every enlightened master, spiritual writer, speaker, teacher, movie star, athlete or diva I have met has feet of clay, inner demons, weaknesses, failures, shortcomings, and blind spots. Most fart and burp and have huge egos or inferiority complexes. Everyone's feet smell when they've worn their shoes too long on a hot day. No matter how far a person evolves spiritually, no matter how wealthy or famous they become, they never stop being tempted by forces that could destroy all they have achieved, or that corrupt their very soul. Our lives progress in spirals, and we all have down times, failures, mistakes, and setbacks, no matter who we are.

"Many advanced spiritual teachers I have held in the highest regard one year have lost their high, pure spiritual vibration a year or two later. Some wear out, burn out, or get lazy; others fall for the lure of easy sex or money and material possessions. Others trip out on power and become insensitive, egotistical dictators; still others fall prey to addictive substances."[16] The history of healing is littered with examples of healers who were seduced by the temptations of the flesh, or lost their way in a maze of sex, money and power. Uma Silbey, author of *Enlightenment on the Run,* advises, "Take the teachings—and run!"[17]

It is essential that a master healer continue her devotion to the divine, even though there may be thousands of people adoring her personally for the healing grace channeled through her. The moment master healers lose the ability to individuate self from patients and fans, they begin their fall from grace. Alice Bailey in her finest book, *Esoteric Healing,* notes that healers often die early of cancer or heart disease.[18] Many unfortunately do not learn the essentials of detachment from their patients, or do not take adequate care of themselves. Ann Nunley, Ph.D. is the originator of an immensely powerful technique for holistic inquiry called Inner Counselor™, which we believe may be the pinnacle of transpersonal healing. Hearkening back to shamanic images of keeping one's spirit pure, she calls the process of self-maintenance "cleaning the bone."

"Once we become enamored with the mask of our own persona we may not be inclined to continue to work steadily and honestly with the substance behind that mask," she observes; "This is why educational programs that focus on spiritual healing should include core courses that teach healers how to stay in touch with elements of their own psychological territory, and methods for consistently addressing and transforming those elements."[19] Intuitive healers graduating from Holos University learn these skills, giving them a life-long skill set that allows them to keep perspective as their ability—and the number of clients they treat—grows.

Consistency

Most of us have brief flashes of healing ability. A mother, when confronted with the sickness of her child, may pray so fervently that the child is healed. During peak states, we may feel a sense of physical well-being that is elevated far above our normal condition.

A master healer has the ability not only to enter the healing space for a few moments, but to hold that space for a prolonged period. Rather than the healing ability of most people, which might flicker on occasionally like a faulty light bulb, a master healer has a practiced ability to turn on the lamp and keep it burning. Master healers know, somatically, in their bodies, exactly what the healing state feels like. They are practiced at entering that somatic condition, just as an athlete knows somatically what condition her body must be in to compete in her sport. Jean Houston, Ph.D., director of the Foundation for Mind Research, the author of fifteen books, and an advisor to UNICEF, says that healers can, "identify with archetypes, and archetypes have the capacity to bring larger patterns of possibility, evolutionary cadences, and a wider spectrum of reality into conscious knowledge and experience." She believes that rapid healing can be the result of the healer "dissolving his or her local self and being filled with an archetypal or sacred image. By bridging oneself between here and the Greater There, one enters into archetypal dimensions that may contain the blueprints of greater possibility, the primal stuff for social and creative change. Archetypal space-time may also contain the optimal template of a person's health and well-being. The job of the healer is to call that template back into consciousness so that it can work upon a malfunctioning body or mind."[20]

That doesn't mean that a master healer is in the archetypal healing space twenty-four-seven. Most require periods of rest and rejuvenation; many thrive on the occasional solitary retreat. But a master healer can consistently enter the healing space, and stay there for long periods of time. Practice makes healing a consistent gift.

Training

Some healers become aware of their ability spontaneously, and train themselves by observing the effects of their thoughts and actions. Others may go through seminary, massage school, a university program in medicine or psychology, or seek another professional credential. We have met several healers who have M.D. degrees, but have chosen to focus on developing their healing powers rather than working within the framework of conventional medicine. And we have met many M.D.s who are healers working within a hospital, clinic, or private practice.

The training of a healer might be in an academic program, the metaphor of learning to which Western culture is most attuned. Or it may be a shamanic apprenticeship, in which a teacher draws back the veil of reality, to allow a student to gain knowledge directly from nature. Pharmacist Constance Grauds tells the following story about her Amazonian teacher, don Antonio, in *Healing the Heart of the World:*

"The shaman's way of healing ourselves and healing the world is done ultimately by creating the Garden of Eden. By creating a Garden of Eden in our lives, we create a positive world, a life-affirming world. ...In this heavenly world of the shaman, all are healthy and have a sense of wellbeing. There is harmony and peace.

"When I asked don Antonio how this might be accomplished, he retorted with his usual answer, 'The jungle itself will tell you.' He then took me on a long walk through verdant jungle trails, knowing that the walk-about experience itself would take me deep into the experience of what he was about to teach me. The answers began unfolding just like the uncurling tendrils of fuzzy green ferns at our feet.

"Don Antonio first instructed me to walk in silence, to experience the jungle without the noise of our human voices. The jungle began to envelope me in an intense, sensurround experience; the squawks of the colorful macaws, the deep calls of the elusive howler monkeys, the green-against-blue shade of the tops of the tall *cecropia* trees reaching the sky. The perfumes of the jungle orchids mingled with the spicy smells of the rotting leaves underneath my feet.

"After some twenty minutes of silent walking, don Antonio whispered to me, 'Tell me what you are experiencing right now.' I answered in a hushed voice, "I'm completely open. I cannot tell if I am breathing, or if I'm being breathed. I am one with everything around me. It is a very heady experience, as if the sense of myself is disappearing. My spirit feels expanded. My heart is so immense that it could fill the universe at this moment. I'm filled with a deep love of myself and everything around me.'

"Don Antonio responded knowingly, 'Welcome to the garden of heaven. The medicine of love is in the sights. The medicine of love is in the sounds. The medicine of love is in the smells. Here, there is nothing but the ultimate medicine of love. From this state of being, all will be healed. You will be healed. From this state of being you will offer to do great things for the benefit of others and the world. I tell you this, for love is the master and you are the servant. Bless you and all the others who have opened your hearts and stepped onto the path of love, for you will now all help to create heaven on earth.'"[21]

Training means different things in different cultures. Jeanne Achterberg, a professor of psychology at Saybrook Institute in San Francisco, senior editor of *Alternative Therapies in Health & Medicine,* and the author of *Rituals of Healing,* emphasizes that every culture has its own metaphors for how the healing process is accomplished. She says, "true, remarkable healing seems to be a function of restoring or reweaving the torn fabric of life in some way. The healee is brought back into a resonant harmony with the community, the planet, and his or her relationships in the broadest fashion imaginable. Rituals appropriate to the situation—pills, potions, chants, surgery, or whatever—seem to be only the visible, technical, and highly variant aspects of healing. The vital factors in the healing process, however, transcend all of these and include intention, motivation, trust, and something as ineffable as passion for living."[22]

Whether the source is the subtle worlds or an academic institution, master healers have sought and completed a training process. One of the most urgent needs in the field of soul medicine is the development of an internationally recognized training program, and accreditation process, for spiritual healers. The work of Holos University is one of the few formal, academically rigorous training programs available in energy medicine. As this field grows, there is increasing demand for an objective standard of competence in soul medicine. Just as medical doctors evolved their own accreditation process a century-and-a-half ago, and chiropractors and acupuncturists a half-century ago, soul medicine practitioners are in the process of evolving an accepted method of identifying adepts in their field.

Section II

The Soul's Historical Primacy in Healing

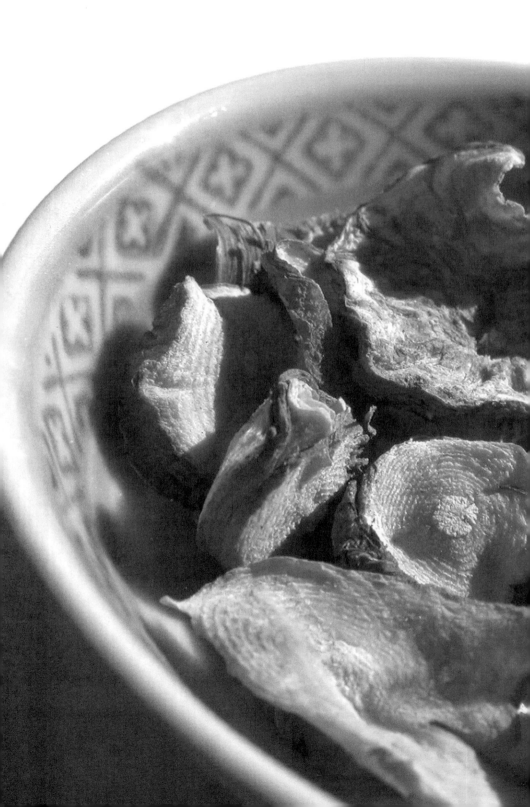

7

Soul, Mind and Medicine in History

Picture, in your mind, walking into a hospital or clinic. You can probably easily imagine a pile of ancient, tattered magazines in a waiting room. You're probably familiar with the scent of antiseptic cleansers on scrubbed walls and floors. You see gleaming metal instruments, bright lights, and elaborate machines. The staff dress in white coats or green scrubs, and may wear surgical masks or caps. Everyone is busy. Pagers, phones, machines and monitors punctuate the background noise of mechanical hum. Newness is everywhere. This is the face of technological medicine, the only medicine with which many Westerners are familiar.

Now imagine walking into a church, or a house of worship. Stillness reins. If there is sound, it is subdued. Soft music designed to soothe and uplift the soul may be heard. Priests and church officers wear the traditional garments of their orders. Ancient rituals, symbols, and hierarchies abound. The scent of well-worn pews and ancient leather hymnals may permeate the air, or perhaps the odor of incense. The whole experience contributes to an atmosphere of reverence.

No one walking into a church imagines that they are walking into a hospital. No one walking into a hospital imagines that they are stepping into a religious sanctuary. Yet this clinical separation of medicine and religion is a recent phenomenon. It was not always so. From the earliest human times, perhaps 100,000 years ago, when trepanning (the boring of holes into the skull) was performed to let out the evil spirits, healing and religion have been intertwined. According to the *Encyclopedia Britannica*, "Many would hold that the most important function of religion has been that of healing—the diagnosis of the cause of evil and mental and physical sickness, and the development of techniques for its cure." *Britannica* goes on to state, "Rarely can a religious leader succeed unless he can heal; no religion has survived that does not heal."

All great religions include healing in one form or another, ranging from blessings and exorcisms to purification. Ritual formulas, prayers and gestures invoke supernatural power; the power of God can protect the devotee and grant everything from health and fertility to the acquisition of wealth. Also, most religions employ charms and amulets, from rosaries to magical mojos, which are blessed in various sacramental ceremonies to perform sacred tasks, ranging from physical protection, to divine guidance.

In many religions, illness is considered to result from behavioral or moral transgressions. The concept of confession or repentance in the face of disease is common. Religious myths speak of gods, heroes and holy people as healers.

The Divine Origins of Disease

Many religious traditions have viewed disease as being caused by deities, demons and devils. Exorcism, purgatives, internal cleansing and surgery have all been recommended as cures for such predicaments.

Some diseases are associated with loss of soul. A specialty of some shamans, especially among Native Americans, is retrieving parts of the soul that are thought to have become dislocated or lost. This process is accompanied by meditation, special magical incantations and ceremonies.

Sinning—when an individual has violated a divine law prescribed by his or her religion—has also been viewed as the cause of illness. In this case, curing comes through confession, repentance, enlightenment or the intervention of a holy healer.

The Bible says that the ancient Israelite King Saul visited a woman at Endor. She materialized the spirit of the great prophet Samuel, who prophesied for Saul. Saint Paul, the founder of Christianity as an organized religion, began his mission after having a vision of Jesus. Though mediums have undoubtedly existed throughout history, human spiritual mediums appear to have achieved widespread acceptance after 1848.

Spiritualism grew out of this mid-nineteenth-century phenomenon. William James, among others, and Gardner Murphy, the great psychologist from the Menninger Foundation, were members of the American Society for Psychic Research. The various spiritualist organizations, ranging from Spiritual Frontiers Fellowship to the Association of Research and Enlightenment, founded by Edgar Cayce and his followers, have emphasized a connection with God and moral principles as the foundation for life. From a spiritualist's perspective, wrong mental (spiritual) thoughts (belief, intent) precipitate disease. The spirit is directly connected with a universal energy called God.

Traditional Healing Practices

Throughout history, the afflicted have sought religious healing in three ways: traveling to a sacred spot (such as one where there is special water to cleanse themselves); consulting a holy person; or obtaining help through a religious object.

Healing Via Water

Springs or temples have typically been the sites to which pilgrimages have been made. Even the Indian Vedic tradition states,

"The waters are indeed healers; the waters drive away and cure all illnesses."

Water is seen as the source of light both in mythology and science. It is also used in physical and psychological cleansing. Hot springs and mineral waters have long been a feature of spas and health resorts. Evidence from the Neolithic and Bronze Ages indicates interest in such spas in France, Italy, and Switzerland associated with religious and healing traditions. In all, several hundred springs and rivers have been considered to have healing powers:

- In ancient Greece, the springs at Chermoplae and Aedepses were sacred to Hercules, the son of Zeus endowed with superhuman strength and courage.

- In ancient Rome, springs at Tibus and hot sulfur springs at Aquae Abulae were well known for their curative properties.

- In the Middle East, Herod attempted to find relief from a fatal illness at in the waters at Callirrhoe, near the Dead Sea in Palestine.

- In ancient Egypt, many of the temples dedicated to the Greek god of medicine, Asclepius, were near or at mineral springs.

The belief that water with healing abilities is charged by a divine presence or a blessing is ancient. Lourdes, in France, is perhaps the world's best-known example. The famous spring achieved its reputation in 1858 after a number of people had visions there of the Virgin Mary. The baths at Scafati, Italy, also contain a shrine to the Madonna. The feast of the Conception of St. John the Baptist is often associated with special healing days. John, of course, baptized his followers by submersion in water.

From ancient times, a belief has existed in the efficacy of certain rivers in restoring fertility to barren women. Civic, church and private religious healing has taken place at many great rivers. The Euphrates river in Iraq, the Abana and Pharpara in Damascus, the

Jordan in Israel, the Tiber in Italy, the Nile in Egypt and the Ganges, Jumna, or Saravati in India have all been associated with purification from transgression, cure of disease and mythical protection into the future.

Healing at Sacred Places

The holy epiphanies are cemeteries or burial places for saints or holy individuals. They are usually surrounded by sacred trees, stones or mountain peaks and are often considered as healing shrines. A good example is the annual pilgrimage to Jerusalem undertaken by many Christians at Easter time. It is interesting that more people go there at the calendar-appointed time of Jesus' death than his birth!

One of the more unusual saints, Saint Rita of Cassea (1381-1456), was reported to have had an incorruptible body. As late as 170 years after her death, Pope Urban XIII viewed the body and reported it to be "as perfect as it had been on the day of her death, with the flesh still of a natural color." About that time, it is reported that her eyes opened and caused a riot! Reportedly, Saint Rita planted a piece of dry wood, watered it each day, and the sticks sprouted into a healthy grapevine, which still bears fruit some 500 years later. The harvest is distributed to high-ranking ecclesiastics. The leaves are dried, made into a powder and sent to the sick around the world. The Blessed Antonio Vici (1381-1461) is another holy figure said to have an incorruptible body. His burial site is reported to have been the scene of miracles of healing.[1]

Holy Healers

A number of monastic orders throughout the world were associated with healing. Some examples are the Knights Hospitalers, the Augustinian Nuns, the Order of the Holy Ghost, the Sorrotes Order and, of course, the Franciscan Order in Europe. Various aspects of the Asclepiads in Greece, the Vomans in India and the Vaidya caste in Bengal also practiced healing. The shamans of many Indian tribes in the Americas have long combined religious and healing practices. Often, healers in indigenous cultures as well as Western civilization trace their knowledge back to the gods.

Perhaps the Franciscan Order has been one of the most successful in maintaining the healing reputation. Many Catholic churches in this country were created by various Franciscan orders of nurses. In the Episcopal church, St. Luke has been the patron saint of hospitals. The Lutheran denomination has also been much associated with hospitals and healing.

Not only priests, kings and holy people have possessed the ability to cure. Ordinary individuals have also demonstrated the special power to heal. Sometimes this power comes on spontaneously in a vision; sometimes it has been sought out by the individual through long periods of meditation, or by mortification of the body. Some of the great religions were founded by individuals with the ability to heal.

There were many well-known Christian healers in the nineteenth and twentieth centuries. Some of them also founded religions or religious organizations. Among them are John of Kronstadt, Furst zu Hohenlohe-Schillingsfurst, Leslie Weatherhead, Edgar Cayce, Oral Roberts, Kathryn Kuhlman, Phineas Quimby, Mary Baker Eddy, Ernest Holmes, and Myrtle and Charles Fillmore.

Mary Baker Eddy founded Christian Science based on Phineas Quimby's work. Quimby, the fountainhead for the entire New Thought movement, focused on healing, and out of that work came First Christian Science. Then came Unity, founded by Myrtle and Charles Fillmore, and Religious Science, founded by Ernest Holmes.

Oral Roberts, at one time a Methodist minister, preached his healing services on radio and television for many years before founding a medical school and hospital in Tulsa, Oklahoma. Katherine Kuhlman, also at one time active in the mainline Protestant Church, offered seminars throughout the country and was accepted even among the most fundamentalist of churches in Springfield, Missouri. Hundreds of people would attend her ceremonies, and those that came forward for healing were often thrown backwards onto the floor when she touched them.

Edgar Cayce has had a wider impact in the field than any other modern alternative healer. Cayce went into trances and did almost 15,000 "readings." Two-thirds of these were related to health, and numerous people attested to healings when they applied the recommendations that Cayce made while in trances. The A.R.E. clinic in Phoenix was founded by doctors Gladys and William McGarry, emphasizing many of the principles first proposed by Cayce back in the 1930s and 1940s. One of these is the use of castor oil, the *Palma Christe* or palm of Christ. It has been demonstrated that a flannel cloth soaked in castor oil and placed on the abdomen with a heating pad will significantly improve immune functions. It is a remarkable palliative treatment for intestinal flu and cramping. Swollen knees also respond extremely well to this particular process. Using the Cayce recommendations, Dr. Gladys McGarry has inspired total recovery in numerous patients from the "fatal" disease of scleraderma.

Spirituality and Religion

Perhaps the most important book ever written in the field of religion and spirituality, *The Varieties of Religious Experience,* was penned by William James.[2] Born in New York City in 1842, the brother of novelist Henry James, William was educated at Harvard where he also taught from 1872 until 1910. He did classical pioneering work in American psychology and philosophy and was regarded as the leading American philosopher of his time.

Although James admitted, "The field of religion being as wide as this, it is manifestly impossible that I should pretend to cover it," it is interesting that he stated, "...the founders of every church owe their power originally to the fact of their direct personal communion with the divine."

The difference between religion and spirituality lies in that statement. Religions tend to establish ritual and dogma to support their particular ideological beliefs. Spirituality is a personal communion

Prayer in the World's Great Religions

CHRISTIANITY:
"When you pray, enter into your closet, and when you have shut the door, pray to your Father which is in secret; and your Father, who sees in secret, shall reward you openly."

CONFUCIANISM:
"Sedulously cultivate the virtue of reverence. When a man is devoted to this virtue, He may pray to Heaven."

BUDDHISM:
"There is no meditation apart from wisdom, and no wisdom apart from meditation. Those in whom wisdom and meditation meet are not far from Nirvana."

HINDUISM:
"I make prayer my inmost friend."

ISLAM:
"Never, Lord, have I prayed to Thee with ill success."

SIKHISM:
"They who cry aloud in trouble obtain rest by prayer and loving God."

JUDAISM:
"Pray to the Lord our God that He may show us the way to go and the thing we should do."

ZOROASTRIANISM:
"He who is called the wise Lord, thou shouldst seek to exalt forever with prayers of piety."

BAHA'I:
"Draw nigh to God and persevere in prayer so that the fire of God's love may glow more luminously in thy heart."

SHINTO:
"If the poorest of mankind come for worship, I will surely grant their heart's desire."

Immortality in the World's Great Religions

JUDAISM:
"The dust returneth to the earth as it was, and the Spirit returneth unto God who gave it."

CHRISTIANITY:
"The gift of God is eternal life, through Jesus Christ our Lord."

ISLAM:
"Those who have believed and done the things which are right, these shall be inmates of Paradise."

JAINISM:
"I know there will be a life hereafter."

CONFUCIANISM:
"All the living must die and, dying, return to the ground, but the Spirit issues forth and is displayed in light."

HINDUISM:
"He becomes immortal who seeks the general good of man."

SIKHISM:
"Why weep when a man dieth, since he is only going home?"

BUDDHISM:
"Earnestness is the path of immortality."

SHINTO:
"Regard Heaven as your father, Earth as your mother, all things as brothers and sisters, and you will enjoy the divine country which excels all others."

TAOISM:
"Life is going forth. Death is a returning home."

ZOROASTRIANISM:
"The soul of the righteous shall be joyful in immortality."

BAHA'I:
"Make mention of Me on earth that in My Heaven I may remember thee."

Peace in the World's Great Religions

CHRISTIANITY:
"Blessed are the peacemakers, for they shall be called the children of God."

CONFUCIANISM:
"Seek to be in harmony with all your neighbors . . . live in peace with your brethren."

BUDDHISM:
"There is no happiness greater than peace."

HINDUISM:
"Without meditation, where is peace? Without peace, where is happiness?"

ISLAM:
"God will guide men to peace. If they will heed Him, He will lead them from the darkness of war to the light of peace."

TAOISM:
"The wise esteem peace and quiet above all else."

SIKHISM:
"Only in the Name of the Lord do we find our peace."

JUDAISM:
"When a man's ways please the Lord he maketh even his enemies to be at peace with him."

JAINISM:
"All men should live in peace with their fellows. This is the Lord's desire."

ZOROASTRIANISM:
"I will sacrifice to peace, whose breath is friendly."

BAHA'I:
"War is death while peace is life."

SHINTO:
"Let the earth be free from trouble and men live at peace under the protection of the Divine."

Love in the World's Great Religions

CHRISTIANITY:
"Beloved, let us love one another, for love is of God; and everyone that loveth is born of God, and knoweth God. He that loveth not, knoweth not God, for God is love."

CONFUCIANISM:
"To love all men is the greatest benevolence."

BUDDHISM:
"Let a man cultivate towards the whole world a heart of love."

HINDUISM:
"One can best worship the Lord through love."

ISLAM:
"Love is this, that thou shouldst account thyself very little and God very great."

TAOISM:
"Heaven arms with love those it would not see destroyed."

SIKHISM:
"God will regenerate those in whose hearts there is love."

JUDAISM:
"Thou shalt love the Lord thy God with all thy heart and thy neighbor as thyself."

JAINISM:
"The days are of most profit to him who acts in love."

ZOROASTRIANISM:
"Man is the beloved of the Lord and should love him in return."

BAHA'I:
"Love Me that I may love thee. If thou lovest Me not, My love can no wise reach thee."

SHINTO:
"Love is the representative of the Lord."

119

Health and Healing in the World's Great Religions

CHRISTIANITY:
"The prayer of faith shall heal the sick, and the Lord shall raise him up."

CONFUCIANISM:
"High mysterious Heaven hath fullest power to heal and bind."

BUDDHISM:
"To keep the body in good health is a duty . . . otherwise we shall not be able to keep our mind strong and clear."

HINDUISM:
"Enricher, Healer of disease, be a good friend to us!"

ISLAM:
"The Lord of the worlds created me . . . and when I am sick, He healeth me."

TAOISM:
"Pursue a middle course. Thus will you keep a healthy body and a healthy mind."

SIKHISM:
"God is Creator of all, the remover of sickness, the giver of health."

JUDAISM:
"O Lord, my God, I cried to Thee for help and Thou hast healed me."

JAINISM:
"All living beings owe their present state of health to their own Karma."

ZOROASTRIANISM:
"Love endows the sick body of man with firmness and health."

BAHA'I:
"All healing comes from God."

SHINTO:
"Foster a spirit that regards both good and evil as blessings, and the body spontaneously becomes healthy."

The Golden Rule in the World's Great Religions

CHRISTIANITY:
". . . All things whatsoever ye would that men should do to you, do ye even so to them . . ."

CONFUCIANISM:
"Do not unto others what you would not they should do unto you."

BUDDHISM:
"In five ways should a clansman minister to his friends and familiars-by generosity, courtesy and benevolence, by treating them as he treats himself, and by being as good as his word."

HINDUISM:
"Do not to others, which if done to thee, would cause thee pain."

ISLAM:
"No one of you is a believer until he loves for his brother what he loves for himself."

SIKHISM:
"As thou deemest thyself so deem others. Then shalt thou become a partner in heaven."

JUDAISM:
"What is hurtful to yourself, do not to your fellow man."

JAINISM:
"In happiness and suffering, in joy and grief, we should regard all creatures as we regard our own self."

ZOROASTRIANISM:
"That nature only is good when it shall not do unto another whatever is not good for its own self."

TAOISM:
"Regard your neighbor's gain as your own gain and regard your neighbor's loss as your own loss."

with God, soul or divine energy. Yet the beliefs of all religions reveal a great deal in common. These similarities were summarized by Dr. Marcus Bach, one of the great mystics and theologians of the twentieth century, in tables on the adjoining pages.

The similarities between the world's religions, on virtually all the great questions of faith, are remarkable. While their external observances may vary wildly, there is almost complete unanimity in their common values. By focusing on those shared values, we may avoid all of the many conflicts that arise from a fixation on the form of worship.

New Thought and Mind-Cure Religions

William James proclaimed that religion is basically a cry for help. This cry for help might take the form of belief in what he called "mind-cures." Mind cures were a logical consequence of the positive theology of the New Thought religions like Christian Science, Unity, Religious Science, and Divine Science. These churches he considered to be "deliberately optimistic," both speculative and practical.

James traced the principles behind mind-cures to a combination of the teachings of the Gospels, to Emersonian or New England transcendentalism, to Berkeleyan idealism, to spiritism, and to Hinduism. Law, progress and development were added to intuitive faith in the healing power of "courage, hope and trust"; "doubt, fear, worry and all nervously precautionary states of mind" were considered harmful.

James went on to state that mind-cures had been observed to heal blindness, lameness and lifelong invalidism. No less impressive were the moral fruits of positive mind-cure belief. James proclaimed that "deliberate adoption" of positive thinking and cheerfulness led to extensive numbers of individuals achieving "regeneration of character." James mentioned as part of the New Thought mind-cure movement the "Gospel of Relaxation" and the benefit of positive affirmations while going through daily routines.

James considered most mind-cure enthusiasts to be pantheistic (the doctrine that God is the transcendent reality of which the material universe and human beings are only manifestations).[3] This movement incorporated the recently "discovered" Freudian-Jungian subconscious into its concept of humankind's intrinsic unity with God. These beliefs aligned it with transcendental idealism, Hindu Vedantism, and Christian mysticism.

James also believed that the development of a personal core of love and harmony, emphasizing positivity instead of negativity, led to greater peace and equanimity, and freedom from anxiety and tension. He emphasizes the "wonder" that this transformation might be the result of simply relaxing. According to James, religion and spirituality provide us with a zest for life, a sense of peace, and a "preponderance" of love, all of which produce "effects psychological or material" in the physical world of our minds and bodies.

During the same century that scientific technology increased the capabilities of modern medicine, the ideas of mind-cure that James described so eloquently developed in parallel, offering people greater serenity, happiness, and the prevention of certain forms of disease. Both science and positive religion led to improvements in health and well-being. In this way, the separation of soul and medicine that began with the Renaissance began to turn full circle. Today, modern research increasingly confirms the vital links between spirit and health. Rather than looking just at ever-improved drugs and surgeries, medicine is reclaiming its ancient roots in healing. The quality of emotional connection between doctor and patient is again receiving attention in medical settings.

When one walks into the building housing the Integrative Medical Clinic of Santa Rosa, California, a scene meets the eye that is very different from the fast-paced, high-tech, scrubbed and impersonal medical setting with which we began this chapter. You check in with a friendly receptionist, then sit on a comfortable couch in a spacious, sunny room with huge picture windows, while waiting for your consultation. You are surrounded by plants and fountains.

A collection of books on healing is accessible in one corner, and an altar provides a quiet focal point for the room. In one corner, there is a play area for children, and a teaching setup for educational classes on enlightened self-care. The open space is used sometimes for movement classes.

You may have a consultation with a highly trained family physician. Alternatively, you may be scheduled for treatment with a nutritional doctor (N.D.), osteopath, psychologist, or somatic therapist. If you receive a prescription, it is as likely to be an herbal formulation as a pharmaceutical drug. If it's a herbal or homeopathic remedy, the medical center has an onsite herbal formulary and kitchen, where your remedy will be prepared. A computer system allows the aromatherapist, psychotherapist or homeopath to determine what diagnosis the medical doctor has made for your condition. Yet the technology can't disguise your sense that a spirit of genuine care and concern pervades each interaction you have in the medical center. You, the whole human being, are the focus of treatment.

Establishments like the Integrative Medical Center,[4] that look completely unlike our traditional ideas of what a treatment center should be, are paving the way for a whole new paradigm of medicine. For the new medical paradigm, soul medicine is a fundamental assumption. It undergirds every aspect of the design of treatment. We don't have to give up the wonders of biomedicine in order to benefit from the insights of complementary and alternative medicine. Science, technology, and conventional medicine are integrated into a treatment regimen that honors the whole human being. As the limitations of the old split become apparent in the collapse of our current "health care" system, science and spirituality are again converging to form a brilliant new synthesis in soul medicine.

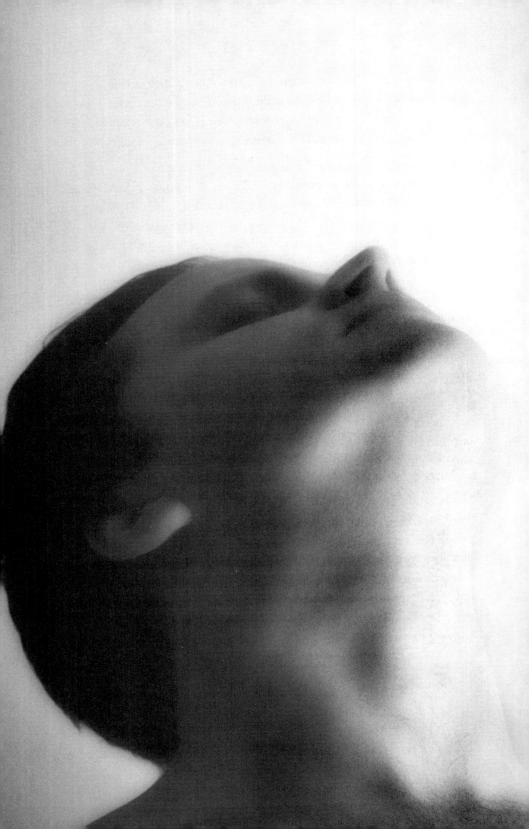

8

Re-Sacralyzing Healing

"**A**rthur's surgery was another middle-of-the-night call, but I got into scrubs in time to walk along beside the gurney as he was wheeled into the elevator and taken down to the fourth-floor operating rooms for cardiac and neurosurgery. ... He went under the anesthetic easily, and before he was draped and the sterile field created, I had time to send energy to his kidneys and to his pericardium by touching points on his feet and hands."

"As Dr. Oz made the incision along the sternum, I leaned over and told Arthur to relax and feel the surgeon's love entering his body. ... When Arthur's heart was out of his chest, I felt in him a sense of abandonment, as if he were a lost child. I reached my arms down under his back to hold him physically and told him to fill the space in his chest with light and energy."

"When the new heart came into the room, I slipped out from my position at Arthur's head and sidled over to the ice chest. Resting my hands lightly on top of it, I acknowledged the heart's fear of the unknown and its sorrow about the death of its old body. Returning to Arthur...I told him that his new heart would make it easier for him to take in love, because he would be able to protect it."

This remarkable account comes from energy healer Julie Motz, and is told in her book *Hands of Life.*[1] She worked initially with patients undergoing heart surgery at Columbia Presbyterian Medical Center in New York with Dr. Mehmet Oz, later author of the best-seller *YOU: The Owner's Manual.*[2] In the course of her work at Columbia and other institutions, Motz was present at dozens of surgeries: masectomies, cardiac procedures, and cancer operations. She sensed the energy of the patient, especially unresolved emotional issues linked to the conditions for which they were being operated on, and helped the patients release the feelings pent up in their bodies. Often the results included instant and dramatic improvements right in the middle of the surgical procedure. Motz is one of the few energy healers who has been permitted in the operating room. Nurses, surgeons, anesthetists, and other staff members had a difficult time adjusting to her presence. There was no institutional role for her, and she was not paid for her work, even though she was clearly having a significant impact on the well-being of the patients with whom she worked. Many members of the medical bureaucracy misunderstood her work, and some actively opposed her.

Yet energy and spiritual work has not always been so separate from medicine. For most of history, medicine and spirituality were inseparable. It is only in our modern era of technological medicine that the presence of an energy healer during surgery might elicit gasps of amazement. For most of medicine's history, the relationship of treatment to spirituality was implicit.

Medicine in Ancient Greece

We consider Hippocrates (approximately 460-370 B.C.), the best-known Greek healer, to be the Father of Medicine. Even in the time of Hippocrates, it appears that scientists who had the greatest political clout had the most influence on medical beliefs in their areas of expertise. For example, Alcmaeon extensively dissected human bodies. He established the connection between a human's sense organs and the brain. He concluded that the brain serves two purposes: it is the "organ" of the mind responsible for thought and memory, and it is a sensation preceptor. A century later, Aristotle vehemently disagreed with Alcmaeon, declaring the heart to be the center of sensation. Aristotle's theory won out and was accepted for many centuries.

At the time of Hippocrates, the Greeks believed illness could be explained in terms of four basic humors: water, air, fire and earth. Each had corresponding qualities: moist, dry, hot and cold. Basic body fluids were believed to be composed of varying proportions of blood (warm and moist), phlegm (cold and moist), yellow bile (warm and dry) and black bile (cold and dry). Deficiency of these humors would cause diseases. Changes in humors could be caused either by external or internal forces.

Treatment generally consisted of diet, exercise and moderation in such habits as eating, drinking, sleeping and sexual activity. Wounds and sores were cleaned and sprinkled with various herbs. Drugs were taken to induce vomiting. Manipulation was used to reduce dislocations and fractures, and techniques for bandaging were extremely well developed. The Greeks used cautery (singeing of flesh) to treat infections, wounds and tumors, as well as the juice of the opium poppy. As part of the diagnosis, there seems to have been an extensive evaluation of an individual's emotional state, habits, surroundings, behavior and customs.

Some seventy-nine books and fifty-nine treatises make up the *Corpus Hippocraticum*. Though the writings are attributed to Hippocrates, a variety of individuals are believed to have completed the work. Of particular note, the treatises insist physicians should look healthy and well nourished, and have a "worthy appearance." Decent clothes should be worn, and the healer was directed to exhibit friendliness. Hippocrates is best known for the Hippocratic Oath:

> I swear by Apollo Physician and Asclepius and Hygeia and Panacea and all the gods and goddesses, making them my witnesses, that I will fulfill according to my ability and judgment this oath and this covenant:

To hold him who has taught me this art as equal to my parents and to live my life in partnership with him, and if he is in need of money to give him a share of mine, and to regard his offspring as equal to my brothers in male lineage and to teach them this art—if they desire to learn it—without fee in covenants; to give a share perhaps of precepts and oral instruction and all the other learning to my sons and to the sons of him who has instructed me and to pupils who have signed the covenant and have taken an oath according to the medical law, but to no one else.

I will apply dietetic measures for the benefits of the sick according to my ability and judgment; I will keep them from harm and justice.

I will neither give a deadly drug to anybody if asked for it, nor will I make a suggestion to this effect. Similarly I will not give to a woman an abortive remedy. In purity and holiness I will guard my life and my art.

I will not use the knife, not even on sufferers from stone, but will withdraw in favor of such men as are engaged in this work.

Whatever houses I may visit, I will come for the benefit of the sick, remaining free of all intentional injustice, of all mischief, and in particular of sexual relations with both female and male persons, be they free or slaves.

What I may see or hear in the course of the treatment, even outside of the treatment in regard to the life of men, which on no account one must spread abroad, I will keep to myself, holding such things shameful to be spoken about.

If I fulfill this oath and do not violate it, may it be granted to me to enjoy life and art, being honored with fame among all men for all time to come; if I transgress and swear falsely, may the opposite of all this be my lot.

Despite the fact that some American medical schools offer this oath, many aspects of modern medicine are in conflict with it.

The idea of sacred healing appears not to have been a part of Hippocratic medicine. The treatises constantly comment about and devote attention to anatomy in great detail. But no actual spiritual connection is noted.

Healing in Ancient Rome

The physician Galen (circa 129-200 A.D.) had a great influence on medicine for about 1,500 years. He reinforced and elaborated on the four fundamental humors mentioned above as the roots of health and illness. Basically, his lasting contribution was to translate the humors into four personalities (phlegmatic, sanguine, choleric and melancholic)—terms still used today. He also dissected extensively, primarily animals and abandoned human corpses. Because he mixed a wide variety of medicinal plants, Galen may deserve recognition as the father of pharmacology.

The introduction of Christianity into the Roman culture gave a strong overlay of religious mysticism to healing. As early as 395 A.D., the Church emphasized healing as being proof of God's grace. Many early hospitals were established by the Church. The Church used numerous icons from its early days in healing ceremonies. Later, the names of various saints—or supposed bits of their bodies or clothes—were also used. The emanations or vibrations from these materials were in themselves believed to initiate healing. Many early Christian writers believed that disease was cured only through prayer and divine intervention.

Christianity extrapolated and incorporated an earlier Judaic principle that disease was a sign of punishment for a sin, or of divine anger. From this religion's beginning, the concept of "the healing mission of Christ" was clearly articulated. In each of the major four gospels of Matthew, Mark, John and Luke (the latter himself a physician), there are numerous instances of Christ acting as a healer in curing paralysis, the inability to speak, blindness, leprosy and fever. Exorcism or "tearing out" of an unclean spirit is also referenced. Throughout the Gospels, no clear-cut differentiation exists between faith healing, exorcism and miracles. The means of healing was always considered to be supernatural. Even in those early days, however, touching was extremely important. Christ often reached out to touch the afflicted or allowed them to touch "the hem of his garment."

St. Benedict, an early Christian saint, actually forbade the study of medicine. That left the concept of divine healing as the only accepted method for about five hundred years. Surgery and pharmacology regressed during this time. Healing practices consisted of prayer, the laying on of hands, exorcism, the use amulets of sacred engravings, holy oil, and the relics of saints. Very little that would be considered either Hippocratic or scientific survived.

The concept that holy individuals could have intercessory powers was fully developed during this period. Indeed, proof that an individual was a saint required the performance of healing miracles. Toward the year 1000 A.D., the intercessory powers of the Virgin Mary also began to be an important part of the healing ritual. To a large extent, Christian healing ignored the scientific discoveries of Greece and the rest of the ancient world.

Ancient Islamic Healing

As the Western world was abandoning the principles established in the Greek and early Roman days, the Islamic world markedly improved the pharmaceutical repertory by developing such methods as distillation, crystallization, solution, supplementation and reduction. Despite these scientific advancements, the Islamic attitude toward the origin of disease remained similar to the Christian idea: Allah caused illness and punished people for their sins. In the Islamic tradition, one could hope for miracles or cures through prayer, and one could also seek divine help through a physician.

Ratzen, a Persian physician and healer, achieved recognition in Islamic culture to a degree similar to that of Hippocrates a millennium earlier. He wrote approximately 237 books integrating earlier Greek medicine into the Arabic world. A Jewish physician, Maimonides, was another healer influential in the Islamic world. Through him and various Arabic physicians, the condition of hospitals was considerably improved, providing better sanitation, care, facilities and medication than Western Christian society had achieved at that time.

The Renaissance and Healing

As the Dark Ages came to an end, Western medicine began to recover, primarily through the establishment of university medical schools. Until about 1500 A.D., folk healers probably treated a far greater number of patients than did physicians or saints. As the Dark Ages merged into the Reformation, surgeons were separated from academic medical practitioners, who held them in disdain.

The concept of medicine as art and science dominated during the Renaissance, with physicians and artists belonging to the same guild. Perhaps the best-known physician of all was the artist Michelangelo. As was common in those days, individuals often had a broad education and might study medicine but not practice it.

During the Renaissance, the average person was more interested in earthly rewards than heavenly rewards. Gradually, control of hospitals and healing transferred from the Church to the City. Physician training began to be regulated and certified. Ideas of contagion and infectious diseases were organized. Public health institutions were established to care for the hopelessly ill and infirm.

However, physicians were not readily available to the general population. In the thirteenth century in Paris, for instance, only a half-dozen doctors served the public. Drugs reappeared and were heavily used throughout the Middle Ages, along with digestive assistants such as laxatives, emetics, diuretics, diaphoretics and styptics.

Mysticism was widespread. Symbolic procedures, such as chants, were widely used. Astrology was believed to play a role in healing. Demons and devils were thought to be causes of illness, and exorcism by a priest was the only prescription. Amulets were commonly used, and various animal parts, especially the genitals, were thought to possess great power.

131

Attempting to wrest control from the Church and saints, royal healers promoted the concept of the king as the great healer, bestower of the royal touch. Bloodletting, which had been popular even in the earliest days, again became widespread in the Middle Ages.

Perhaps the most famous Renaissance physician was Paracelsus (1493-1541), or Theophrastus Bombastus von Hohenhein. A Swiss physician, he was interested in various mystical and occult sciences and was extremely hostile toward his contemporaries. He believed the influence of the stars and planets upon the "astral body" of the patient was the major cause of disease.

Paracelsus is credited by many for creating modern medicine when he proposed substitutes for the concepts of Galen, which had dominated the profession for so long. He went back to the Hippocratic Corpus. His blending of theological and popular thought integrated mysticism and neoplatonism, and urged a new way of knowing. Jan Baptista van Helmont sought to give form and dimension to Paracelsus's cosmology. During the same period, Frances Baker also established an "alternative path to knowledge of nature."

A French physician, Ambroise Pare, became the leading surgeon of the time. He initially insisted on treating gunshot wounds with boiling oil. Fortunately, he found that it was less efficacious than simple debridement of the wound. He reintroduced cautery, and the use of ligatures (tying off) on bleeding blood vessels.

The Scientific Revolution and Healing

When the Scientific Revolution began in the 1600s, people started asking how instead of why things happen. At this time, the major medical treatments were bleeding, purging, dietary restrictions, exercise and the use of various herbs and minerals. Any aberrant medical activity was considered to be "witchcraft." A most important drug, quinine, was introduced for the treatment of malaria.

Toward the end of the eighteenth century, electricity was introduced to medicine, and during much of the nineteenth century various and sundry electrical apparatuses influenced the practice of medicine.

The advent of science did much to discourage or displace the earlier practices of sacred healing, the royal touch, laying on of hands, prayer, and so on. Scientific advances in the twentieth century have virtually wiped out reliance on mysticism, saints and sacred healers. Despite this, the failure of drugs and surgery to cure many illnesses, especially chronic ones, has allowed some institutions and "old ways" to remain popular. For example, Lourdes maintains its attraction for those seeking miraculous healing. Folk medicine and various forms of laying on of hands and therapeutic touch continue to be passed down through generations, enjoying a revival of sorts today. And the stream of research studies, books, television shows, and magazine articles at the junction of spirituality and medicine today bears ample testament to the beginnings of the return of the soul to medicine.

While in many previous eras, scientific medicine and soul medicine were in conflict, today they are allies in healing. Science is gradually demonstrating the principles and mechanics behind those forms of spiritual healing that are effective, while soul medicine increasingly turns to science to identify the most reliable and consistent methods of healing.

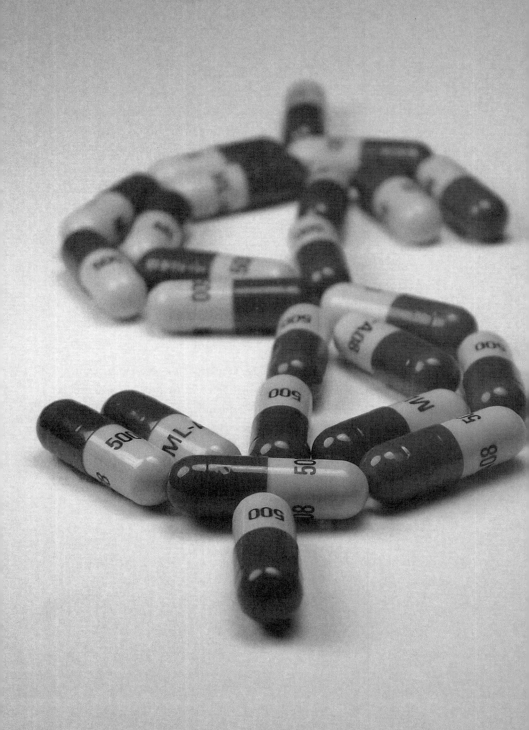

9

Sparking Spirit's Healing Flame

A revival of faith in soul medicine is sweeping Western society. In a 2003 poll, *Newsweek* magazine reported that, "84 percent of Americans said praying for others can have a positive effect on their recovery. Fifty–three percent say they've personally relied on religious faith to help them get through a major illness or health problem. A full 72 percent of all those polled believe God can cure people given no chance of survival by medical science."[1] These numbers are echoed by a cover story in *Time*[2] magazine, reports in *USA Weekend* magazine,[3] and many other popular periodicals. The largest and most comprehensive study done to date, reported in 2005 by the National Institutes of Health, surveyed some 31,000 American adults. It found that 36 percent of them had used complementary and alternative medicine (CAM) in the preceding twelve months. But when prayer was included in the definition of CAM, the figure rose to 62 percent.[4] Soul medicine is becoming part of the fabric of medical care and public awareness to a degree not seen for five centuries.

Why this resurgence in a primordial belief that science rejected hundreds years ago? One reason is the impersonal nature of modern science and medicine. "Managed care," modern medicine's inadequate answer to financial pressure, does a barely adequate job of *management*, and a poor job of *care*. Another reason is the failure of modern medicine to fulfill its promises. Larry Dossey, a respected author and physician, states in his book *Prayer Is Good Medicine* that 80,000 Americans die each year because of infections acquired while in the hospital. This is about twice the number of Americans killed in automobile accidents a year, and more than died in either the Vietnam or Korean wars.

The *Journal of the American Medical Association* has been warning about the seriousness of this problem for over a decade, publishing research showing the dangers of infection, injury and death in American hospitals.[5] One of its careful studies, performed by Dr. Barbara Starfield of the Johns Hopkins School of Hygiene and Public Health, logged:

12,000 deaths due to unnecessary surgeries

7,000 medication error deaths

20,000 deaths due to other errors in hospitals

80,000 deaths due to infection

106,000 deaths due to non-error, negative effects of drugs.

Deaths totaled some 250,000 patients in a year. Bear in mind that these numbers are just for deaths; they don't include patients getting sick from similar causes and recovering, or suffering temporary or permanent impairment due to medical treatment.[6]

These studies rank iatrogenic or doctor-caused illnesses among the largest killers of Americans, right up there with heart disease and cancer. Other studies, with different criteria, actually find that iatrogenic illnesses are the number one killer. A meticulous analysis of data from U.S. government studies found that, in 2001, heart disease killed 699,961 people, and cancer killed 553,252 people—while the conventional medical establishment dispatched some 783,966 patients. The cost to society is estimated to be $282 billion dollars a year.[7] Researchers have macabre arguments about whether to rank iagtrogenic illness the number one, number two, or number three killer. But no-one disputes the seriousness of the problem.

Furthermore, complications from drugs and surgery are the reasons for one-third of patients being admitted to critical care units. "In any other sphere of modern life, this situation would rank as a national scandal," says Dr. Dossey. Compared with prayer, "Modern medicine would win the death derby every time by a landslide."[8]

Dr. William Nolen, in his book *Healing, A Doctor in Search of a Miracle,* stated that healers can cure 70 percent of individuals—a statistic that appears far better than the average drug.[9] Scientific proof indicates that soul medicine is at least as good as most drugs. Virtually no single drug is as effective as soul medicine. Astonishingly, the U.S. Congress, Office of Technological Assessment, has reported 85 percent of the drugs now in use have no satisfactory scientific documentation backing them.

Some of the established drugs are not as safe as the frequency with which they're used would lead us to assume. A study published in *New Scientist* in December of 2005, performed by William Lee at the University of Texas Southwestern Medical Center in Dallas, caused a furor. It found that acetaminophen, the active ingredient in Tylenol and many other over-the-counter painkillers, is the leading cause of acute liver failure in the U.S. Nearly half the deaths attributable to liver failure after consuming acetaminophen were accidental overdoses. The study followed comatose patients suffering liver failure. According to the journal, "of the 275 people with acetaminophen poisoning, 8 percent received a liver transplant, 65 percent survived without one and 27 percent died." Some of the patients had overdosed unintentionally, taking two or more prescriptions that they were unaware both contained acetaminophen. But patients who overdosed themselves deliberately, and were quickly treated, had similar degrees of liver damage.[10]

Despite millions of dollars spent by pharmaceutical companies on finding and promoting new drugs, very few effective new treatments come to market. According to the most comprehensive study ever conducted of anti-psychotic drugs, expensive new pills are no more effective, or safer, than old ones. Funded by a $44 million grant from the National Institutes of Mental Health, conducted by Columbia University psychiatrist Jeffrey Lieberman for publication in the *New England Journal of Medicine,* it found that the new class of drugs called atypical anti-psychotics, a market worth $10 billion a year to drug companies, is no more effective—or safer—than perphenazine, an old generic drug. Perphenazine, largely discontinued because doctors routinely prescribe the new drugs, is one-tenth the cost.[11]

Lieberman points out that 90 percent of drug trials that appear in the scientific literature are funded by drug companies. There has been evidence that drug companies suppress publication of clinical trials that are unfavorable to their drugs, such as discontinuing studies when early results are unpromising. According to the *Washington Post,* "the industry has recently come under fire for hiding unfavorable trial data."[12] Two huge studies of antidepressant medications released by the US federal government in 2006 also demonstrate that the most commonly prescribed medications "failed to show that the drugs were safer or more effective than a placebo."[13]

Britain's respected *Independent* newspaper, in its "Science" section, under the headline, "Glaxo Chief: Our Drugs Do Not Work on Most Patients," reported that: "A senior executive with Britain's biggest drugs company has admitted that most prescription medicines do not work on most people who take them.

"Allen Roses, worldwide vice-president of genetics at GlaxoSmithKline (GSK) [a huge multinational drug company], said fewer than half of the patients prescribed some of the most expensive drugs actually derived any benefit from them.

"It is an open secret within the drugs industry that most of its products are ineffective in most patients but this is the first time that such a senior drugs boss has gone public. His comments come days after it emerged that the NHS [Britain's universal health service] drugs bill has soared by nearly 50 percent in three years."[14]

According to an article in the *Seattle Times,* entitled "The Hidden Big Business Behind Your Doctor's Diagnosis," and written by a respected medical reporter Susan Kelleher, "some of America's most prestigious medical societies take money from the drug companies and then promote the industry's agenda."[15] The result? "Millions of people taking drugs that may carry a greater risk than the underlying condition. The treatment, in fact, may make them sick or even kill them."[16] Franz Ingelfinger, the late editor of *The New England Journal of Medicine,* once said:

"Let us assume that 80 percent of patients have either self-limited disorders or conditions not improvable, even by modern medicine. The physician's actions, unless harmful, will therefore not affect the basic course of such conditions. In slightly over 10 percent of cases, however, medical intervention is dramatically successful.... But, alas, in the final 9 percent, give or take a point or two, the doctor may diagnose or treat inadequately, or he may just have bad luck. Whatever the reason, the patient ends up with iatrogenic problems. So the balance of accounts ends up marginally on the positive side of zero."[17]

Or perhaps on the negative side of zero, when we consider the financial and ethical costs of allopathic medicine as it is currently practiced. In a 2006 editorial entitled "Seducing the Medical Profession," the *New York Times* says, "Last week two new cases came to light that reveal the lengths to which companies will go to buy influence with doctors, pharmacists and other medical professionals. Reed Abelson reported in the *Times* on Jan. 24 about a whistle-blower's lawsuit alleging that Medtronic had paid tens of millions of dollars in recent years to surgeons in a position to use and recommend its medical devices. In one particularly egregious example, a prominent Wisconsin surgeon received $400,000 for just eight days of consulting. In last Saturday's *Times,* Gardiner Harris and Robert Pear revealed that a Danish company paid a pharmacist, doctors' assistants and a drug store chain to switch diabetic patients to the company's high-priced insulin products." The *New York Times* concludes that, "The critical issue is that doctors must have the best interests of their patients at heart in prescribing drugs or recommending medical devices. Their judgment must not be clouded by financial self-interest or the desire to please industrial benefactors."[18]

A 2006 report in the *Journal of the American Medical Association* examines the many incentives given by drug companies to physicians to prescribe their products.[19] Gifts, trips, consulting contracts, ghostwriting services, meals and samples are showered on doctors by pharmaceutical manufacturers in an attempt to sway their decisions. The amount is not trivial. It is estimated to be $19 billion in an article in *USA Today*.[20] By way of comparison, that is *double* the dollar volume of the entire retail book industry—*all* the books sold at retail in an entire year in the United States. "Marketing ... should not be allowed to undermine physicians' commitment to their patient's best interest or to scientific integrity," the authors of the report write, recommending that such gifts be banned. "Research in the psychology and social science of gift receipt and giving indicates that current controls will not satisfactorily protect the interests of patients," they conclude.

Soul medicine is poised for a comeback as the preferred means of primary medical care. It should always be the treatment of choice when orthodox medicine has nothing to offer. It should also serve as an ancillary treatment even when surgery and drugs are indicated as necessary. As Olga Worrall once said, "Another little touch of healing never hurt anyone." A century ago, Sir William Osler, the father of American medicine, wrote eloquently of the importance of faith in health and healing:

"Faith is the great lever of life. Without it, man can do nothing; with it, even with a fragment, as a grain of mustard seed, all things are possible to him. Faith in us, faith in our drugs and methods, is the great stock in trade of the [medical] profession.... As Galen says, confidence and hope do more good than physic— 'he cures most in whom most are confident.' That strange compound of charlatan and philosopher, Paracelsus, encouraged his patients 'to have a good faith, a strong imagination, and they find the effects.' While we doctors often overlook or are ignorant of our own faith-cures, we are just a bit too sensitive about those performed outside our ranks. We have never had, and cannot expect to have a monopoly in this panacea, which is open to all, free as the sun, in which may make of everyone in certain cases, as was the Lacedemonian of Homer's day, 'a good physician out of Nature's grace.' Faith in the gods or in the saints cures one, faith in little pills another, hypnotic suggestion a third, faith in a plain common doctor a fourth. In all ages the prayer of faith has healed the sick, and the mental attitude of the Suppliant seems to be of more consequence than the powers to which the prayer is addressed. The cures in the temples of Aesculapius, the miracles of the saints, the remarkable cures of those noble men, the Jesuit missionaries, in this country, the modern miracles at Lourdes and at St. Anne de Beaupre in Quebec, and the wonder-workings of the so-called Christian Scientist are often genuine and must be considered in discussing the foundations of therapeutics. We physicians use the same power every day.... We enjoy, I say, no monopoly in the faith business. The faith with which we work, the faith, indeed, which is available today in everyday life, has its limitations. It will not raise the dead; it will not put a new eye in the place of a bad one...nor will it cure cancer or pneumonia, or knit a bone; but in spite of these nineteenth-century restrictions, such as we find it, faith is a most precious commodity, without which we should be very badly off."[21]

Whether a doctor or a soul medicine practitioner, the healer who assists the belief or faith of a patient may accomplish more than any drug of surgery! If they can channel grace, even more so. Only those patients requiring life- or function-saving medical or surgical intervention—probably no more than 15 percent of patients—need drugs or surgery to help them. Surgery or drug intervention should always be considered in cases of serious diseases, such as major infections, fractures, certain types of cancer curable by surgery, and congestive heart failure.

An extremely wise professor of medicine, Eugene A. Stead, Jr., advised that a physician should primarily serve as a triage officer.

When a patient first comes in with a complaint, the role of the physician is to verify that there is no serious illness that requires immediate medical or surgical intervention. If the patient is not suffering from a potentially serious illness, then he or she should be presented with various forms of healing and allowed to *choose* the modality or modalities. Indeed, the physician should even consider stepping aside to preclude the patient becoming worse off.

Drugs and surgery are inappropriate for many chronic illnesses, especially those representing stress reactions without measurable physical dysfunction. This is most true for depression, anxiety and panic attacks, and all of the psychoneurotic and neurotic illnesses. Even for chronic illnesses, where drug therapy could improve quality of life for diabetes or congestive heart failure patients, it is always appropriate to complement or supplement those therapies with a safe alternative. For instance, insulin certainly may be required in diabetes, but the addition of chromium picolinate, 1000 micrograms per day, and vanadium 50-100 micrograms per day, might enable a patient who develops diabetes after age thirty-five to reach a point where insulin isn't needed. And there is certainly evidence in some patients that soul medicine can diminish diabetes.[22] Potentially beneficial forms of soul medicine to consider in such cases include acupuncture, transcutaneous electrical nerve stimulation, hypnosis, biofeedback, creative imagery, osteopathic manipulative therapy, chiropractic therapy, improved nutrition, Reiki, attunement, therapeutic touch, massage, homeopathy, light and color therapy and aromatherapy. Any of these approaches can invite the patient's soul into the treatment.

Soul Healing Practices

There are many healing modalities that work with a patient's energy, facilitating its flow, and removing blockages to soul expression through body, mind and emotional realm. Some of them are:

1. Meridian-Based Therapies

Acupuncture, the oldest therapy based on the body's energy

Shamanism (Brazil, Africa) has also demonstrated some remarkable healing powers.

12. Prayer, and Faith Healing

Prayer and intercession for the sick is one of the oldest forms of healing on record. It can establish a direct connection between the soul and the ailing body. Faith healing is included here because most faith healers use intercessory prayer to request healing for the sick.

13. Conscious Lifestyle

Conscious exercise, conscious eating, meditation, relaxation and other healthy lifestyle changes are a deliberate choice that reclaims personal responsibility for wellness. A conscious lifestyle is one in which a person makes decisions that promote healing and soul connection, living an outer life in harmony with the soul's expression. A conscious exercise routine may include yoga, dance, or the martial arts.

14. Subconscious Reprogramming

Researchers remind us that, while our conscious mind processes some 400 bits of information per second, our subconscious mind processes upwards of eleven million bits per second.[28] The information contained in our subconscious can thus override the best of conscious intentions. Affirmations, muscle testing, and other therapies that influence the subconscious mind attempt to clear from messages that get in the way of soul healing.

Attitude and the Nature of the Sacred

Our state of consciousness, our choice of relationship to the divine, is under our control. It is ultimately consciousness, and our attunement to the divine, that instill health, nurturing, love, and a desire to do good. A positive, cheerful, optimistic attitude and self-motivation are as important as diet and exercise in determining health and healing.

Consider the following characteristics of a limited human

personality, the column on the left. Compare it to the characteristics of a soul expressing through a body, mind and heart, on the right. When our attitude is one of soul awareness, linked to the benefits of soul medicine, we unlock our full potential as spiritual beings on a human path.

Limited Personality Nature	Soul Nature
negativity	joy
pessimism	optimism
materialism	holism
pride	dignity
need for authority	intuitive knowing
desire	detachment
self-deception	enlightenment
intolerance	acceptance
separatism	unity
cruelty	benevolence
arrogance and selfishness	nobility
prejudice	tolerance
impulsiveness and impatience	patience
laziness	motivation
destructiveness	productivity
stubbornness	flexibility
inconsistency of direction	creative purpose
fearfulness	courage
anger	peace with serenity
resentment	forgiveness
hatred	love and goodwill
jealousy	trust
self-pity	resourcefulness
guilt	self-respect
possessiveness	magnanimity
victimization	empowerment
reactiveness	self-determination
rebellion	harmony and cooperation

greed	charity
sexual profligacy	sexual-spiritual attunement
hedonism	restraint
irresponsibility	responsibility
judgmentalism	discernment
resignment	endurance
ugliness	beauty
untruthfulness	honesty
uncertainty	faith
dogmatism	wisdom
annoyance	broad-mindedness
mental rigidity	abstract thought or reason
taking offense easily	impartiality
focus on the past	focus on the present
self-absorption	responsiveness to spirit
competition	cooperation

All of these are stressful and involve sympathetic activation, increased adrenalin, a loss of magnesium, and exhaustion.

All of these are restorative; parasympathetic, and may activate homeostasis effect through subtle quantum states of well-being.

In the next chapter, we'll take a closer look at how to cultivate the qualities of the soul in everyday life, and by doing so, how we can unlock the huge benefits that flow from communion between soul, heart and body.

SECTION III

Quantum Healing

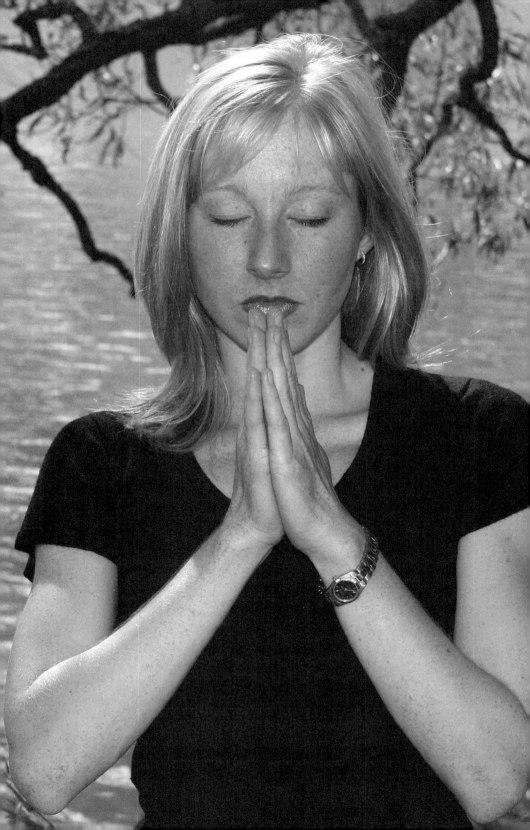

10

Your Personal Soul Connection Inventory

By now we hope we've convinced you that paying attention to your spiritual life is the most important thing you can do for your health. A healthy relationship with your soul, and using soul medicine as primary care, is the best thing you can do for your body. In this chapter, we'll talk about some of the specific characteristics of a strong soul connection, and give you a chance to measure your spiritual practice against a set of criteria that many authorities believe indicate a vibrant relationship between soul, heart, mind and body.

Evelyn Underhill, a great Christian mystic, stated that spirituality is not living in a monastery or nunnery. It is the attitude you hold in your mind when down on your knees scrubbing the steps.[1] Indeed, it is the right approach to life whether engaging in menial work or facing the greatest of personal tragedies. Viktor Frankl, the great Austrian psychiatrist, felt that a sense of meaning was the single most critical factor in surviving the unbelievable atrocities of a German concentration camp, including abuse, starvation and even typhus infection.

Today, spirituality is considered an important part of secular life. No longer is it necessary to cloister oneself to invoke the sacred. We are surrounded by a growing chorus of personal-growth groups, books, tapes, men's movements, women's movements, and youth movements. Many of these groups are attempting to fill the void that has occurred in the last fifty years since the relative breakup of extended and nuclear families. Society is responding to its existential crisis by seeking meaning.

Even though technology has partially trivialized the transcendent and organized religions have lost members, while society has tumultuously and radically changed, strong spiritual countermovements have arisen and may become proportionately stronger as the mechanistic view of evolution pushes the envelope of affluence, if not of influence.

Concomitant with the spiritual decay of the Vietnam War, the redeeming influence of the humanistic psychology movement was born. It was followed by the transpersonal psychology movement, and then the holistic health and medicine movement. Humanistic psychology emphasized the importance of the individual, of feeling, of self-actualization; of what Carl Jung called individuation—the movement of the individual toward ultimate adult maturity. The transpersonal psychology movement emphasized a connectedness with spirit, soul, and God. The holistic health movement emphasized the importance of the spiritual aspects of life in overall well-being. Today, soul medicine works with energy in direct new ways, bypassing many of the deliberative protocols of talk therapy and even holistic health modalities.

The Power of a Soul-Conditioned Consciousness

What is spirituality? Charles Fillmore, founder of Unity, in his book *The Twelve Powers of Man*, emphasized twelve faculties that he felt represented spirituality: faith, strength, discrimination or judgment, love, power, imagination, understanding, will, order, zeal, renunciation, and life energy.[2] Fillmore was one of the first to attempt to define spirituality; many later writers have given their own definitions, and our understanding of the nature of spirituality continues to expand. For instance, we are indebted to Dean Ornish for laying out so eloquently and convincingly in his book *Love and Survival* how closely linked a sense of community is to both spiritual and physical health and longevity.[3] "Community" did not appear in Fillmore's list, but no modern list would be complete without it.

How do we apply the principles of spirit to health? As we contemplate the nature of the soul, and seek to integrate its attributes into our everyday thoughts and actions, we support good health. Below is a list of characteristics we have found to be common to people with a vibrant soul connection, wherever and however it may be practiced. A connection with your soul can be deliberately cultivated as part of a healthy life:

1. **Forgiveness**: The most important single attitude required to initiate the healing process is forgiveness. Carrying a grudge is like taking poison yourself—and expecting it to kill your worst enemy. Letting go of the negative thoughts that we have harbored is the first step in the healing journey. Until we release and forgive, we anchor ourselves to our negative experiences, and continue to reap the consequences of our attachment. Forgiveness means giving up our stories, our justifications, our recitals of how badly we've been treated, our victim stance, and stepping into the bracing air of personal responsibility, where love, grace and serenity wait to guide us on our healing journey. When we identify with soul, we can do nothing other than forgive, because holding grudges is simply not part of the soul's nature.

2. **Tolerance**: Acceptance of human differences, beliefs and behaviors, without being judgmental, is the essence of tolerance. Tolerance does not condone harmful actions by or toward other people. But it keeps an open mind to seeing things from the other's point of view. A soul viewpoint sees all viewpoints, and is not stuck in narrow human interpretations.

3. **Serenity**: Serenity is ability to be at peace, especially when there is turmoil around you. Serenity is the result of trust in a benevolent universe, and gives us the strength to remain steadfast through our life's challenges. Serenity implies a trust in the steadfast and unchanging nature of the soul, rather than having ones consciousness dominated by the passing show of what the Hindu scriptures call *maya,* the illusory visible world. Charles Fillmore refers to the serenity of David, who trusted in God to overcome the enormous physical power and size of Goliath. Serenity knows that there is a source of spiritual power far beyond the apparent balance of force in the world. Serenity allows us to remain present in the moment, rather than being drawn into fears of what might happen, and of having our minds consumed by negative imaginings. Serenity stays rooted in the real, and in the parts of reality that we can influence, rather than agonizing about the parts we can do nothing about. Serene people are resilient, able to remain intact and grounded when problems arise. Serene people bring themselves back to this calm place when they find themselves out of it; they have well-developed practices they use to cultivate an unshakeable soul connection in the midst of a busy, distracting, and disturbing world.

4. **Faith**: Faith is the ability to maintain the belief that life moves always in the direction of our good. Faith places greater emphasis on the reality of an immortal soul and a benevolent universe than on the transient reality of a perishable body. As an example, Charles Fillmore discusses Abraham, who was willing to sacrifice his son Isaac under the direction of God, even though he did not understand why God would make such a request. He mentions many other biblical examples, such as the fall of the walls of Jericho. The Israelites acted under the direction of a power higher than any material calculation of military strength, and witnessed a miraculous victory as a result.

5. **Reason**: When he talks about reason, Fillmore is referring

to spiritual understanding or spiritual illumination. Spiritual grounding results in the ability to look honestly at conditions, without being mislead by our conditioning or the chatter of our minds. Understanding is the ability to penetrate below the surface appearance of the world, and, from the soul's perspective, grasp the greater spiritual principles at work. It involves detachment, allowing us to apply logic and rationality to the problems before us, rather than reactivity. This dispassionate discernment allows us to choose the best solution for all concerned, the soul's aim of the "highest good of all." As an example of enlightened reason, Fillmore cites Solomon, who chose wisdom above riches and honor. Judgment, discrimination, intuition and inner knowing are all aspects of wisdom. Reason guides us into wise choices, rather than knee-jerk emotional reactions to people and situations. Reason keeps us present in time and space, rather than wandering constantly into the realm of imaginary fears and projected outcomes. Reason enquires into the values, motivations and lifestyles of others, rather than staying stuck in a provincial spiritual or material culture.

6. **Hope**: Hope is the expectation that the future will be better. Hope is the ability to imagine a better tomorrow, and use the human imaginative capacity to create images of increase and success. Early in the twentieth century, the autonomic nervous system was called "the imaginative nervous system" because it was known that imagery affects the function of the body, and through proper imagery, regeneration can occur. Hope is the belief that grace flows freely. Webster's dictionary defines grace as "charm, elegance, attractiveness, especially of a delicate, slender, refined, light or unlabored kind...unconstrained and undeserved divine favor or goodwill, God's loving mercy displayed to man for a salvation of his soul." In religious terms, grace implies complete acceptance and forgiveness by God, whether we deserve it or not. Grace is an aspect of God's unconditional love. Grace can result

in healing or rescue that completely defies explanation or reason. It just *is*. Hope is the expectation of grace.

7. **Motivation**: Motivation is the inner drive to accomplish worthwhile things with our time on Earth. Motivated people have confidence, and believe in themselves. Motivated people find the places within them that contain the strength to face their obstacles. Motivated people use their will to express and pursue their needs and desires. When the barriers between the earthly facilities of mind, body and heart are removed, and the soul expresses freely, it brings great power, will and motivation to the earthly incarnation.

8. **Consistency**. Having the strength of intention and commitment to undertake a regular spiritual practice is a foundation of the spiritual path. That could mean weekly church attendance, or daily meditation. When you ask a group of regular meditators how long it took them to enter a state of meditation easily, you may hear answers ranging from ten years to fifty years. The difference between a person who can enter that state at will and one who can't is that the former person has stuck with their practice, however inconvenient, boring, difficult, or unsuccessful it seems at times. Charles Fillmore talks of power, dominion, and mastery: He's not referring to physical dominion, but to the mastery that comes only from consistent spiritual practice. Identification with the soul results in a consistency of spiritual practice and enlightened behavior. Cultivating frequent soul contact results in consistent expression of soul qualities.

9. **Community**. Solitary hermits have sometimes attained enlightenment, and there is a rich tradition in most religions of placing oneself apart from the world in order to focus on spiritual understanding. However, such a vision quest is usually of limited duration, after which one reenters the world. Moses heard the Ten Commandments on top of Mount Sinai, but they would have been no use to the people of Israel

unless he had come down from the mountain and led them in applying the Commandments in daily life. Retreats and grail quests are a vital part of the spiritual search, but ultimately, we express our spirituality communally. Spiritual community is also a magnificent support system to help us maintain our practice when it seems most difficult. The Buddha described the *sangha,* the community, as one of the "three jewels" in which we may take refuge on the path to enlightenment. Recent research suggests that a rich social network makes an enormous difference in health and longevity. Humans may differ in everything, including their religious views. An old saying goes: "Where you have one Dutchman, you have a church. Where you have two Dutchmen, you have schism." Yet the soul perceives a unity beyond human differences. When Jesus was offered the Roman coin by his enemies, who knew that he could be condemned no matter which of the two options he picked, he confounded them by choosing a "third order" solution that saw the unity beyond the apparently opposing answers. The soul sees community where the brightest human minds see only differences.

10.**Joy**: Joyful people are an inspiration to those around them, and a blessing to the world. Joyful people appreciate and express the beauty in life. They cultivate a sense of happiness by appreciating and expressing the beauty in life. They are determined to find the positive in every situation. A deeply spiritual life, lived in the abundance of God's grace, leads inevitably to joy. Communion with the divine illuminates the inherent joy in oneself and in the world; out of the overflow of the joyful heart, lightness and contentment spring. Joy is automatic in a soul-generated life.

11.**Gratitude**. Any inquiry into the nature of life leads inevitably to gratitude. The miracle of physical life, and the confluence of divine presence with material existence, naturally lead the spiritual person to give thanks. A person with a strong spiritual foundation wakes up with gratitude for the opportunity for soul to express into the world, and reawakens to gratitude whenever he or she contemplates the state of grace in which we live. Most people are grateful for obvious blessings such as unforeseen gifts, money, the birth of a child, a holiday, or a great accomplishment. By contrast, the soul is rooted in gratitude as a state of being, thankful to the creator in each moment for the magic and majesty of life. Grateful people give thanks for mundane, everyday events such as a meal, water, or a good night's sleep; they don't need an extraordinary display of grace to evoke feelings of thankfulness. Living from soul, gratitude becomes a way of approaching each day, rather than an occasional event-based feeling.

12. **Love**: Love has many aspects. Love is the unconditional desire to aid others. Fillmore believed that unconditional love is not a preference; it is "the desire to do good to others." Love includes compassion, a deep sense of empathy toward those who are suffering misfortune or undergoing personal trauma. Love includes charity, the desire to share time, energy, wisdom and money with others. Love means not necessarily *enjoying* nurturing others without conditions or reward—but *desiring* to do so nevertheless. Unconditional love—without judgment, with no need to know why—is a cornerstone of the Christian faith. It is often regarded as the ultimate nature of God and the soul. A person anchored in their soul is anchored in love.

Soul Connection Inventory

How do you perceive your own experience of these twelve aspects of spirituality? The following quiz is designed to test your application of these attributes. Score yourself on the following scale, for each item below. Write down the first score that comes to you, rather than taking a lot of time to think about your answer. Then add up your scores to get a sense of the areas of your spiritual life in which you need support, and the areas in which you have mastery.

5. I Strongly Agree

4. I Agree

3. I'm Neutral

2. I Disagree

1. I Strongly Disagree

1) All things work together for good.

2) God is benevolent.

3) I have a soul that survives death.

4) My life on Earth is meaningful.

5) Once a week or more, I reverently watch a sunset, sunrise, or natural scene.

6) I meditate, pray, or think about the beauty of life regularly.

7) I feel calm and serene when things go wrong.

8) I can face whatever life offers.

9) I have sometimes wronged or harmed others.

10) I have apologized when I've wronged others.

11) I can learn from my problems and mistakes.

12) I am wise enough to make the right choices.

13) My spiritual beliefs change as I understand more.

14) I set reasonable standards and goals for myself.

15) During the course of my life, I have read three or more books about a religion other than my own.

16) I helped someone within the last week.

17) Service to others equals service to God.

18) I tithe regularly.

19) In the last year, I have contributed to help others in misfortune.

20) When I see a person or animal in pain, I feel that pain.

21) I am connected to all living beings.

22) I go out of my way to help other people.

23) Tomorrow will be better.

24) Miracles happen.

25) Human beings can change their ways and improve themselves.

26) I usually forget wrongs that have been done to me within a few days.

27) I send blessings to people who have wronged me.

28) I send myself love when I've done something I wish I hadn't.

29) When I hear a belief that differs from mine, I consider it deeply.

30) I defend the right of others to have their beliefs, different from my own.

31) Religions other than mine may contain wisdom for me.

32) When someone acts badly towards me, I try and see their point of view.

33) When I become frustrated, I pause and calm myself.

34) I can accomplish anything to which I apply myself.

35) I am able to keep focused even when other people don't believe in me.

36) I have a consistent daily spiritual practice.

37) I read religious or inspirational materials at least once a week.

38) I pray once a week or more for myself and others.

39) I believe that my attitude each day is more important than attending church.

40) I sent a blessing in my thoughts to someone else in the last two weeks.

41) I have a trusted spiritual advisor.

42) I have two or more close friends.

43) I worship weekly at a church or spiritual center.

44) I said "I love you" to two or more people in the last week.

45) I gave someone an unexpected gift in the last month.

46) I often spontaneously feel great joy in my life.

47) I deliberately look for things to be happy about each day.

48) Every morning I'm thankful just to wake up.

49) I give thanks to God whenever good things happen.

50) I give thanks go God whenever bad things happen, even though I may not understand why.

Interpreting Your Results

Add up your scores. A score of 200 or more indicates a strong and robust spiritual life, with a heart and mind congruent with soul values. A score of 150 to 200 indicates that soul and consciousness have a strong connection, yet there are areas of your spiritual practice that need strengthening. A score of 149 or below means that you need seriously bolster your spiritual life. To find which of the twelve areas require specific attention, take a look at your responses again. Questions 1 through 4 relate to your attitudes and practices concerning *faith*. Here are how the other groups of questions are structured:

5 through 8 measure your application of *serenity* and your ability to *live in the moment*.

9 through 15 measure your application of *reason, honesty, wisdom* and *understanding*.

16 through 22 measure your practice of *love, compassion* and *charity*.

23 through 25 indicate your sense of *hope* and belief in *grace*.

26 through 28 measure how practiced you are at *forgiveness.*

29 through 33 show your degree of *tolerance* and ability to be *non-reactive.*

34 and 35 show your application of *will,* and your degree of *motivation* and *confidence.*

36 through 40 indicate how diligently you *apply* yourself, and how *consistent* you are.

41 through 45 measure your sense of *community.*

46 and 47 indicate how much *joy* you express.

48 through 50 measure your sense of *gratitude.*

For a copy of the quiz broken into areas of spiritual practice, see the endnotes.[4] Please don't feel bad about a low score in any area. Take it as feedback, and a gentle nudge to pay attention in that area. The simple act of bringing consciousness to an endeavor is often enough—alone—to catalyze change. This scoring instrument draws from several other indices of spiritual well-being, but is a quiz rather than a thoroughly tested scientific instrument. It's meant to help you notice the areas that are strong and weak in your spiritual practice, rather than being a definitive assessment of how you behave. Celebrate the strong areas of your spiritual expression, and recommit to them, for the health of both your body and your soul. Talk to a guide, minister, coach or friend about the areas in which you're weak, and come up with a plan to support your soul in pouring vibrantly through you in every way. Your body will love you for it!

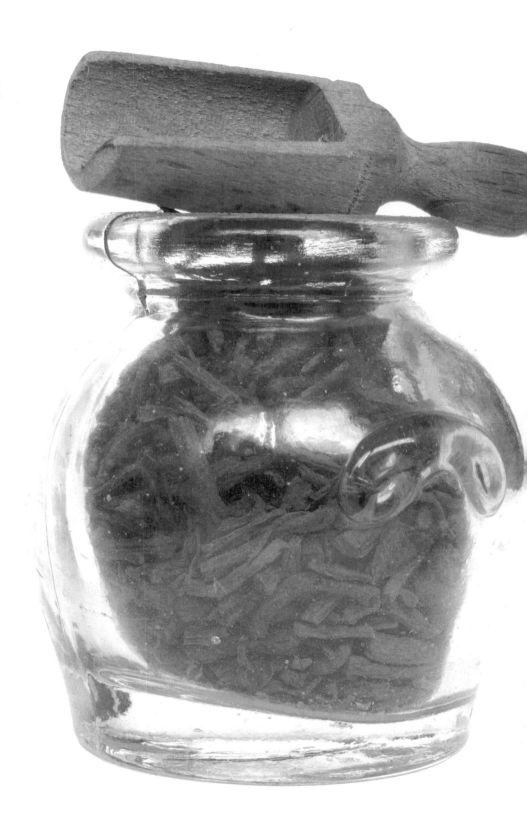

11

Soul Medicine as Primary Care

To most patients, the simple relief of their symptoms is adequate proof of a cure. Unfortunately, for many illnesses, a cure is more difficult to prove scientifically. An understanding of the foundation for scientific proof is crucial to grasping the remarkable nature of sacred healing.

From a physician's point of view, very few illnesses have enough scientific documentation to prove that they are physical illnesses. A fractured bone is clearly a physical illness. It usually takes six to twelve weeks for the healing of a fracture. If a healer could lay on hands and cause the bone to heal within two weeks, that would "prove" effectiveness. Medicine generally believes that type I or childhood diabetes—diabetes that begins before age thirty-five—is not reversible, and that the patient will require insulin throughout his or her life. When the onset of diabetes occurs after age thirty-five, it is often controllable by diet, physical exercise, and even deep relaxation training—though many physicians still do not offer these alternatives and just put the patient on drugs, at most suggesting dietary control.

It would be difficult for sacred healing to "prove" cure of a type II adult onset diabetic, whereas reversal of type I would be dramatic. Cancer is perhaps the most dramatic illness. "Spontaneous" healing of cancer is indeed a very rare event. Thus cancer above all other illness offers the best opportunity for proof of healing. Nobel laureate Albert Szent-Gyorgi said, "Do we understand cancer? No, nobody does. Our real problem is not 'What is cancer,' but 'What is life?' We can't understand cancer until we understand life, because cancer is just distorted life."[1]

Allopathic Explanations

What is real or genuine? Hypertension or high blood pressure is perhaps a prime example of the dilemma in medicine. Most physicians would admit that hypertension is to some extent the result of stress, and yet stress reduction is rarely recommended adequately or taught. For many years it was believed that sodium was the major culprit in hypertension. There is now some evidence that chloride may be more important than sodium. It is also now known that almost all hypertensive patients are deficient in calcium and even more deficient in magnesium. But these replacements are rarely recommended by physicians. Instead, they prescribe drugs that usually (after a trial of several different drugs) will bring the patient's blood pressure under control. Such drugs often cause complications, ranging from increased risk of suffering a stroke, to the loss of sexual potency in men. Drugs offer, at best, a standoff-they: can control the blood pressure—but at a significant psychological and physiological cost.

Dr. Elmer Green at the Menninger Foundation, who introduced temperature biofeedback for the control of migraine headaches more than three decades ago, demonstrated that 80 percent of hypertensive patients could bring their blood pressure under control with temperature biofeedback. His results have been sustained for over two decades, and yet many physicians deride biofeedback as merely a "placebo." An 80 percent success rate is hardly a placebo, and the control of hypertension with biofeedback is genuine, but because this treatment does not enrich drug companies, it has not been publicized to the medical profession. Such are the philosophical dilemmas in medicine today.

In the medicinal community, there is virtually never total agreement on either diagnosis or therapy, even within the same school of thought. The conflict between allopath and holistic medicine is even greater.

For example, Andrew Taylor Still, an M.D., introduced osteopathy in the late nineteenth century. He attempted to have it accepted at the University of Kansas, which had been founded by his family members. But his concept that abnormal position, particularly of the vertebrae, produced pressure on arteries and resulted in dysfunction that could be corrected by manipulation was soundly rejected by the medical profession. Osteopaths were treated almost as contemptuously as were chiropractors by allopaths until the mid-1960s, when the AMA suddenly agreed to accept osteopaths as being equally trained and offered osteopaths the opportunity to drop their D.O.s and become M.D.s just with the stroke of a pen. Some 2,000 did so, but most retained their osteopathic roots.

Homeopathy is even more controversial than osteopathy. Samuel Hahnemann (1755-1843), a German physician, introduced homeopathy at a time of "uncertainty, contention, and contradiction" as one German medical professor called his age. Hahnemann was quite disillusioned with many of the medical practices of his day, which included leeching, bloodletting and purging. He introduced substances to healthy individuals and made a detailed record of the symptoms they produced. He then diluted those substances many thousands or millions of times to treat patients whose symptoms were identical with the symptom pattern developed when that substance was administered in larger doses. Hahnemann called this the law of similars, that is, like cures like. In allopathic practice, drugs are used to control or suppress the symptoms of an illness. In homeopathy, extremely dilute amounts of the substances that "cause" the symptoms are given to desensitize or strengthen the body's inherent healing ability. Allopathy supports the law of opposites; homeopathy promotes the law of similars.

Allopathy—with an emphasis on drugs and surgery—has dominated scientific medicine for a century. Other remedies have been rejected, attacked, criticized or legally suppressed. The oldest forms of soul medicine, including acupuncture, nutrition, sacred healing, herbs, massage, and manipulation, have received short shrift from the medical profession.

The Placebo Effect

Logical, systematic, and mathematical principles are the basis of conventional medicine. Proof of efficacy and safety are accomplished by double-blind, crossover research studies. Double-blind means that neither the patient nor the therapist knows what the patient is receiving. Generally, one-third to one-half of the patients are given a placebo (a sugar pill or an injection of distilled, sterile water), and the other half or two-thirds are given what is thought to be the "active" drug. The purpose of this approach is to prove that a given treatment is statistically more likely to improve a specific symptom or physical condition to a greater degree than a placebo would accomplish under the same circumstances.

In cross-over studies, after an initial treatment period ranging from one week to a month or more, the subjects who received placebo receive the "real" drug, and those who received the drug now receive the placebo. Again, neither the physician or nurse dispensing the medication nor the patient knows whether the patient is receiving placebo or an "active" drug. Theoretically, this allows any differences between the two to become more apparent, and proves the degree to which the drug is more effective than the placebo. Placebos typically average 35 percent effectiveness. A difference of only a few percentage points is taken as proof that the drug is superior to the placebo. Drugs must succeed by only 2 percent more, or 37 percent, to be considered therapeutic if the 2 percent superiority is consistent in a few thousand patients.

Double-blind studies are tedious and difficult to conduct. One needs to look at many different factors, not just a single symptom. Results are subject to hundreds or thousands of variables. For instance, in looking at hypertension, smoking, caffeine intake, sugar intake, calcium, magnesium, body weight, genetics and physical exercise are all variables that can influence blood pressure significantly. In fact, these same variables are virtually equally important in affecting diabetes. And there is, of course, individual biochemical variability. Some individuals metabolize carbohydrates easily; others have trouble with many carbohydrates, not just simple sugars but even starches. "Jack Sprat could eat no fat; his wife could eat no lean" is folk wisdom for a real medical distinction. Blood cholesterol and triglycerides are also affected by many different factors, including sugar intake, caffeine, nicotine, alcohol, exercise, weight and genetics.

Dr. Herb Benson, a Harvard internist, demonstrated in 1979, through rigid scientific study, that no treatment of angina pectoris, either by drugs or surgery, was better than the 35 percent placebo effect.[2] But physicians who believed in their treatment reported an astounding 90 percent success rate. (The remaining 10 percent of people failed to respond, which is true in the best of cases.) Absolutely no pill or surgery safely achieves that success, including coronary bypass surgery and all the drugs used for angina. The physician's belief—and indeed the patient's belief and intent—is the factor most dramatic in determining healing.

Dr. Bruce Moseley, a surgeon practicing arthroscopic surgery at the Baylor College of Medicine, enrolled patients in a study designed to discover the relative value of two kinds of surgery that are used as treatment for osteoarthritic knees. One, debridement, scrapes away damaged cartilage. The other, lavage, flushes out the site. Both types of surgery are done through small incisions made on either site of the kneecap. The study was published in the *New England Journal of Medicine* in 2002.

To control for the placebo effect, a third group of patients received only a pretend operation, instead of the real thing. During the placebo operations, patients were anesthetized, incisions were made, the staff shuffled around the operating theater for the average amount of time it took to perform a real lavage or debridement, and the incision was then sewn up. Absolutely no surgery was done on their knees.[3]

In a series of follow up examinations over the course of the two years following surgery, the difference in results between the patients who had received the actual surgery and the placebo became apparent. It was approximately *zero*.

In television interviews, some of the patients who had received the placebo operation swore it must have been real, because their knees were so dramatically improved. Some reported the cessation of pain, or a vastly increased range of motion. Some who were barely able to walk before surgery were now able to run. Not only had the patient group receiving the placebo experienced recovery rates similar to those who had actually received arthroscopic surgery; at certain points in the recover process their reported results were better. Dr. Moseley, the researchers, and his staff were astounded. There are 650,000 arthroscopic debridement or lavage procedures performed in the US each year. Each one costs some $5,000.[4] The total cost is over three billion dollars per year.

We believe that this threshold of proof, just a few percentage points higher than a placebo, is not worth the many problems and side effects of most drugs and surgery. If a drug is twice as effective as a placebo, with limited and acceptable side effects, then it is reasonable to consider it as a therapy. The threshold at which drugs are considered effective needs to be raised dramatically.

Western medicine has emphasized X-rays, blood chemistry analyses, and electrocardiograms as diagnostic tools. Neurologists and neurosurgeons have often relied on electroencephalograms (EEG). Computerized analysis of EEGs can now measure differences of less than 1 percent between the two sides of the brain, and document them with graphic color pictures. Increasingly, such "brain maps" are becoming accepted by the medical profession, especially among those who are experienced and well read in this subject. Blood tests, which are relatively stable, are also another good test of therapeutic effectiveness. DHEA, the most ubiquitous hormone in the human body, is reported in scientific literature to be very stable, changing not more than 15 percent at various times of day or with different seasons. Thus a change of 25 percent, 50 percent or 100 percent in DHEA concentrations is scientifically remarkable. Tests can show the effect of various therapies on DHEA levels.

The placebo effect is powerfully at work in all surgeries. Loren Eskenazi, a plastic surgeon and professor at Stanford University, writes in the recent anthology *Consciousness & Healing:* "Just as in an initiation rite, wherein the initiate is removed from outer life and is cleansed with smoke, water, blood or other means, we ask our patients to fast and to cleanse themselves with antibacterial soap the night before. The initiate is stripped naked and redressed in ritual garments, and our patients must take off their street garments and wear a special, albeit humiliating, hospital gown. Initiates often engage in an elaborate procession to the temple, church, or sacred ground where the ceremony occurs, and surgical patients kiss their loved ones goodbye and walk down a long hallway and enter the sacred space of the 'operating theater.' Like the initiate, they willingly lie down on a table, which is the altar upon which the transformation occurs. As most cultures use trance dancing, drumming, or soma (mind-altering drugs) to induce altered states, surgical patients surrender to anesthesia...undergoing a symbolic death and rebirth upon awakening. Surgery is a modern blood ritual enacted for the purpose of healing. After an operation, the community witnesses the scar and knows that the individual has been forever changed."[5]

The placebo effect is as much at work in soul medicine as any other therapy, and future studies will control for it. When a sacred healer is able to produce a documented cure, such as the cases we have listed, this is demonstration of their efficacy—especially where drugs and surgery have failed. A clue as to why soul medicine can be effective for so many different conditions comes from professor

Helen Graham of Keele University, who writes, "A person can be given exactly the same inert preparation and, depending on the label given to it by the doctor, can convert it into a beta blocker, stimulant, anxiolyic, antidepressant or anti-cancer drug. Given such a substance and told that it is a painkiller, a person will produce painkilling effects.... The same inert substance, when used to treat ulcers, may be converted into an H2 receptor blocker.... When given to treat high blood pressure, the same substance may be converted into a specific molecule—a beta blocker—that could not be more different. A patient given such a substance as an anti-cancer treatment may find that his or her hair falls out and the gums begin to bleed. What this means is that in each case a person converts a belief into a very specific molecule, that is, a very different biochemical reality, which in turn produces a very different physiological result. So-called miracle cures can be effected in this way."[6]

One of the most exciting potential tools for studying the effects of soul medicine is the DNA microarray. DNA microarrays are pieces of silicon, glass, or plastic to which lengths of specifically designated DNA segments are attached. Thousands of different DNA segments, called reporters, can be attached to a single microarray. The microrray can be used to study changes in gene expression that occur, for instance, during different stages of a disease. DNA microarrays have the potential to stimulate research that identifies how gene expression changes before and after soul medicine treatments.

These scientific tools are now available to study the effects of soul medicine, and over the next decade we expect to see a large number of new studies that demonstrate its effectiveness in conventional scientific terms, in addition to the studies already performed, some of which we refer to in this book. For the last half-century, these measurements have been used primarily by drug and surgery practitioners to validate their therapies; they are now increasingly demonstrating the effectiveness of soul medicine and other non-invasive therapies.

The Danger of Drugs

Drugs can produce a remarkable variety and range of side effects or even serious complications. For every drug included in the *Physicians' Desk Reference,* the list of complications, adverse effects and warnings is enough to scare the stoutest heart. These side effects can be minor problems or major illnesses. Drugs may cause both a drop in well-being, as well as severe sickness. Dizziness, agitation, insomnia, drowsiness, constipation and diarrhea are among the most common symptoms. They may occur spontaneously, with no clear-cut "cause," and without a major ailment. They may occur with placebos as well as with drugs.

With most drugs, these particular symptoms are only slightly more common than they are with placebos. On the other hand, most mood-altering drugs, such as antidepressants and tranquilizers, and most cardiovascular drugs (those used for hypertension or other heart disorders) have a much higher incidence of these common symptoms—as well as more serious ones. The major reason that dizziness, agitation, insomnia and so forth are so common is that those are symptoms associated with stress. Mental and emotional anxiety can easily produce those particular symptoms. Mood and cardiovascular drugs work to alter the stress response; thus they may add significantly to the natural background stress level. In general, these relatively common symptomatic side effects are not serious or life-threatening.

But because there are safer, less disruptive alternatives, why use drugs as a first course of therapeutic action? Which is the more sensible and ethical treatment: a placebo with a 35 percent effectiveness and no side effects, or a strong drug with 39 percent effectiveness and dramatic effects on the patient's sense of well-being? Because placebos work as well as many drugs, and alternative medicine often works better, society is due for a major rethink of its drug addiction.

When Allopathic Medicine Works Best

The crowning achievement of allopathic scientific medicine is the ability of M.D.s to make a specific diagnosis. Congestive heart failure, diabetes, hypertension, and various forms of cancer are easily diagnosed. Although remarkable advances in surgery have been made in the last two centuries, such procedures would be unusable without proper diagnoses. Truly miraculous diagnostic tools are available today, such as MRI (magnetic resonance imaging), enabling detailed evaluation of the brain, spinal cord and many other organs with a clarity often beyond that which is visible even surgically. Allopathic diagnostic capability is truly superb.

Once a diagnosis is made, and even with advanced drugs and surgical therapy, just how good is modern medicine compared with holistic medicine?

In general, allopathic medicine is particularly good in treating acute illness—and not so good at treating chronic illness. Acute illnesses include significant injuries, serious infections, fractures and shock. Chronic illnesses include cancer, rheumatoid arthritis, lupus erythematosus, osteoarthritis, multiple sclerosis, diabetes, emphysema, asthma, congestive heart failure, chronic pain, migraine and stroke. Allopathic medicine is also minimally helpful in curing chronic hepatitis, stroke, retinitis pigmentosa, macular degeneration, allergies, chronic fatigue syndrome and depression. There is also new evidence that some conditions previously labeled as "psychiatric" may in fact be autoimmune diseases; researchers have recently found ways in which even anorexia and bulimia demonstrate the hormonal characteristics of autoimmune disease.[7] The degenerative diseases may also be helped by the general improvement of a patient's energy systems through alternative medicine. Degenerative diseases may be the result of energy blockages and the loss of cooperation among the subtle energy systems of the whole network of life. These conditions can be improved only by energy medicine. In the words of researcher James Oschman: "In the past it had been thought that the genes give rise to proteins that then spontaneously assemble into the living structures that carry out living processes, including consciousness. In the emerging quantum model, it is the action of quantum coherence that organizes the parts into living structures, and it is the action of quantum coherence that gives rise to consciousness as a distributed and emergent property of the assembled parts."

Though symptom control clearly can often improve a patient's quality of life, that is the only remedy conventional medicine offers for most chronic illnesses. It does not offer a cure. Regardless of allopathic medicine's most advanced cancer treatments, 50 percent of patients still die within five years from many types of cancer. Chemotherapy can destroy or radically diminish the quality of a patient's life. A recent analysis of twenty-five years of breast cancer records from all over America by doctors at the Sloan-Kettering Cancer Center showed that, for all its cost, complexity, misery, and pain, the most significant improvement in breast cancer treatment may be nothing more elaborate than early detection.[8] If surgery or antibiotics cannot cure a problem, safe alternatives are preferred if they either cure, or improve the patient's quality of life.

Stress & Health

Hans Selye (1907-1982), the brilliant physician who introduced us to the concept of stress, discovered a correlation between health and stress in the nineteen-thirties. Thousands of scientific papers have documented the multifaceted face of stress in both minor disease and serious illness. Essentially, they show that when there is enough pressure—physical, chemical, emotional or electromagnetic—to cause a doubling in the amount of adrenaline in the blood, then blood sugar goes up, increased insulin is produced, and a stress response occurs. Selye called this "an alarm reaction."

If one is exposed to the same stressor repeatedly, after a short period of time the stress reaction does not occur. This is the stage of *adaptation*. Selye emphasized, however, that every time one adapts to a stress, the threshold for new stress is lowered.

Even sub-threshold amounts of stress are cumulative. For

instance, it takes one cigarette to raise adrenaline production to roughly twice the normal level. A third of a cigarette has very little effect. It takes a cup of coffee to produce an alarm reaction. But one third of a cup of coffee, a third of a cigarette and two teaspoons of sugar together produce an alarm reaction. Eventually, individuals begin to "burn out." This is the stage of *maladaptation* which, according to Selye, is a feature common to all significant illnesses. And eventually, when the body cannot cope at all, a terminal state occurs, which Selye called *exhaustion*. Yet despite the ubiquitous role of stress in disease, stress reduction is rarely a part of allopathic treatment.

The Effect of Belief and Intention

Early in the 1900s, Emil Coue, the French pharmacist, was cited by European physicians as having cured tens of thousands of patients. He accomplished this through a simple positive affirmation, "Every day, in every way, I am getting better and better." Although Coue's work is generally derided, a placebo's power may be stronger than any drug or surgery because it represents an individual's belief. Mocked by the American Medical Association, Coue may still have the last laugh.

During the last two decades, psychoneuroimmunology has become a major new science. It is now known that the immune system is more powerfully influenced by attitude and belief than virtually all other normal factors combined. While a patient's belief is a key factor in his or her healing, sacred healing can also take place without the patient's knowledge or participation. Absent healing is as enigmatic as grace to healing. The healing occurs without an individual knowing of an interdiction by way of prayer or a sacred healer. Convincing evidence of the efficacy of absent healing by prayer has been demonstrated in a study of patients in the cardiac care unit. In a double-blind study, without the patients' knowledge, half of a group of patients had absent prayer directed toward them while the other half did not. Those who received absent prayer had a statistically significantly greater survival rate and a shorter hospital stay. Those persons for whom there was no specific group prayer did not do as well.[9] These results might have been even more striking if we knew whether those who did not receive the group prayer had families praying for them or were intervening in their own way with prayer. In other words, some of the controls may have done better because of unreported prayer assistance.

Edgar Cayce, one of the most quoted intuitive diagnosticians of all time, often stated that physical illnesses were the result of unsatisfactory attitudes. "No one can hate his neighbor and not have stomach or liver trouble. No one can be jealous and allow the anger of same and not have upset digestion or heart disorder" (Reading 4021-1). Another of his almost 15,000 intuitive readings states, "Hate, malice, and jealousy only create poisons within the minds, souls, and bodies of people" (Reading 3312-1). He pointed repeatedly to the fruits of the spirit—love, kindness and patience—as essential to health.

There are so many documented cases of belief affecting healing that choosing from among them is difficult. The *Baltimore Sun* newspaper looked at studies that showed clinical effects from patients' beliefs,[10] and summarized some examples:

- Patients who were taken off blood-pressure medicine for three weeks so they could try a new drug saw their blood pressure drop to normal in the period when they were taking no drug at all.

- Thousands of elderly Chinese Americans in California born in years with bad astrological qualities died sooner from cancer than Chinese Americans with the same disease who were born in good astrological years. A study of whites with the disease revealed no similar correlation of cancer deaths and astrological signs in birth years.

- A saline injection was enough to kill the pain in 30 to 40 percent of people who got their wisdom teeth out, according to one study at the University of Maryland. A symbolic injection stimulated patients' production of morphine endorphins in a twenty-year-old California study.

- In a classic 1958 study, patients underwent sham surgery for angina (pain due to a constricted blood supply). They got local anesthesia and were cut slightly, but they did better than patients who actually had the surgical procedure.

Patient belief has been dramatized in series of articles published by University of Connecticut psychologist Irving Kristol, Ph.D. A 1999 study of his caused an uproar in the psychiatric community. He examined nineteen studies, and found that at least 75 percent of the effect of any antidepressant drug—yes, that's *any* antidepressant drug—you take your pick—was caused by the placebo effect.[11] A patient's belief represented three quarters of the effect. And possibly more; antidepressants make you *feel* different, while sugar pills don't. So a portion of the remaining 25 percent may be due to the physical sensations induced by the drug, and thus also due to the placebo effect—or, as the American Psychological Association puts it in their abstract of Kristol's article: "These data raise the possibility that the apparent drug effect (25 percent of the drug response) is actually an active placebo effect."[12] Though officially double blind, meaning that patients theoretically had no idea whether or not they were on an active medication, in practice the studies were "unblinded," since the side effects were often sufficient to demonstrate to those on the medication that they were in the experimental group and not the placebo control group.

Not content with the furor stirred up by his earlier heresy, Kristol recently published a meta-analysis of the FDA database of 47 studies of the six most commonly prescribed antidepressants. He included "file drawer" studies—those aborted by their sponsors (usually drug companies) for "failing" to produce any discernable effect by the drug being studied. These studies are well worth including. For a drug to be approved, the FDA requires that it be shown to be more effective than a placebo in at least two clinical trials. This sometimes results in many clinical trials being conducted before two positive results are obtained. One reporter observes that "the efficacy of Prozac could not be distinguished from placebo in six out of ten clinical trials."[13]

He found that an average of 80 percent of the effect of the drugs was due to the placebo effect. This ranged from a low of 69 percent (Paxil) to a high of 89 percent (Prozac). In four of the trials that Kristol studied, the placebo exhibited better results than the drug. The mean difference between the placebos and the drugs was a "clinically insignificant" difference of two points on the Hamilton Depression Scale.[14]

Kathy McReardon, one of the subjects involved in one of those studies of antidepressants had suffered from severe depression for years, and made a number of suicide attempts. Her depression had frayed her marriage and deeply affected her ability to parent her son. After receiving the placebo, her depression disappeared. She knew she was participating in a study, and after the trial ended she was told that she had received the placebo. So strong was her belief that she had received the trial drug and not the placebo that she went back to her psychiatrist and insisted that a mistake had been made. She was absolutely convinced she had received the new antidepressant drug that was the subject of the trial.

The doctor checked. Kathy was wrong. She had only received a sugar pill. Nevertheless, she had been cured. A follow up two years later showed that her depression had not returned despite her discovery that she had been given a placebo. Television footage of her with her family before the study shows a person who is barely recognizable compared to the happy group shown afterward.

It is safe to assume that the placebo effect is as active in recipients of prayer as it is in recipients of Prozac. The effect of a patient's belief is as strong in the case of soul healing as it is in mechanistic medicine. Yet while there are far fewer studies of soul interventions than there are of conventional medical practices, the studies that are available often indicate large effects, much larger than the 10 to 20 percent efficacy typical of a study of a drug or surgical procedure. Studies of soul medicine keep revealing what researchers call "big effects" or "big data" such as the dramatically shortened recovery times for prayer recipients described in previous chapters.

It will be interesting to see the day when trials of drugs are routinely performed side by side with studies of prayer, healing touch, directed intention, acupuncture, and other modalities of soul medicine.

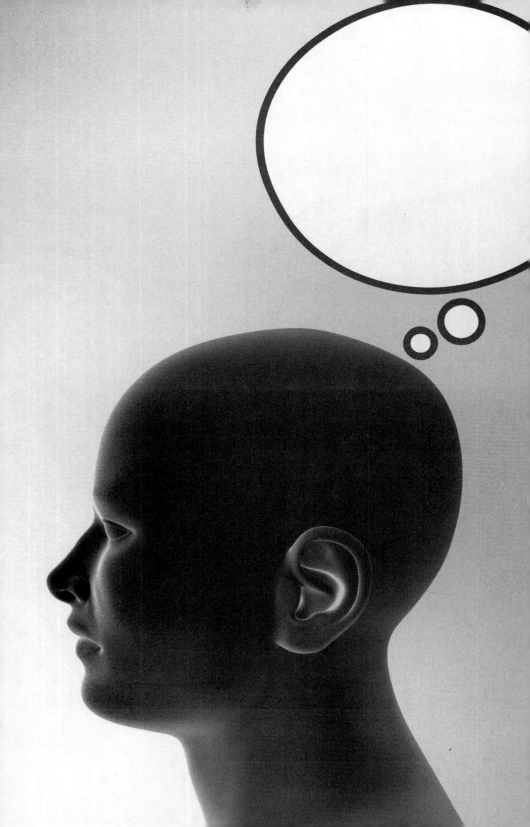

12

A Quantum Brain in a Neuroplastic Universe

For years, the placebo effect was considered to be a purely psychological mechanism. New brain research has shown that it is the opposite; that a patient's beliefs stimulate the brain to manufacture a wide variety of biochemicals. In one study published in *New Scientist,* fourteen healthy young men were given a medication that, they were told, "may or may not relieve pain." They were then given injections in their jaws that produced pain. The researchers then measured the production of the body's natural opiates, the endorphins. Brain scans revealed that after the subjects took the placebo, their brains released more endorphins. This means that there is a measurable physiological change occurring, not just a psychological effect.[1] In another study that reinforces the physical realities that occur in our bodies in response to a belief, 148 British college students were given fake alcohol. They were served in a bar, and believed they were drinking real alcohol like those around them. When tested, they showed some of the same types of impairment the genuinely drunk students demonstrated. "When students were told the true nature of the experiment at the completion of the study, many were amazed that they had only received plain tonic, insisting that they had felt drunk at the time,' the researcher commented, concluding that, 'It showed that even thinking you've been drinking affects your behavior.'"[2]

A number of years ago Norm Shealy's six-year-old son was overheard talking with another six-year-old. The visiting child said, "My father is a cardiologist. He is the most important doctor because the heart is the most important organ."

Norm's son, Brock, replied, "My father is a neurosurgeon and the brain is more important because the brain controls the heart."

The conflict the children raised is not a new one. Debate about both the seat of the mind and the dominance of heart or brain has been going on for at least two thousand years. Indeed, to a greater or lesser extent, a major theme throughout philosophy has been an ongoing debate about the mind. Benjamin Rush (1746-1813), physician, patriot and signer of the Declaration of Independence, wrote extensively on the moral faculty as "a power in the human mind of distinguishing and chasing good and evil" in a lecture given at the American Philosophical Association's Annual Oration in 1786. Rush made a strong distinction between moral action and moral opinion of conscience. He attempted to show the physical causes such as the size of the brain, heredity, disease, fever, climate, diet, drink and medicines all could affect the mind's moral ability.

Joseph Buchanan (1785-1829), physician, educator, inventor, lawyer and journalist, published in 1812 *The Philosophy of Human Nature*, perhaps the most original contribution to American psychology prior to William James. Buchanan was probably the first to articulate the Law of Exercise in which he stated that every action becomes more common in reaction to the frequency of the stimulus and that repetition increased "the excitability" of the brain. Amariah Brigham (1798-1849), a psychiatrist, published in 1832 his *Remarks on the Influence of Mental Cultivation upon Health*. Fear was growing at that time that the complexity of "modern" life would increase the incidence of insanity!

Throughout the nineteenth century, there was a widespread perception of a disorder called *neurasthenia*. Florence Nightingale, the founder of modern nursing, suffered from that disorder, which included several dozen physical and mental symptoms, ranging from insomnia to hypersensitivity, as well as pain, irritability, and depression. It was generally considered to be a "functional" disorder rather than a psychological one. At the end of the twentieth century, health professionals began to have considerable discussions about a similar disorder commonly called Chronic Fatigue Syndrome (CFS). Patients with CFS often present numerous neurological, chemical and biochemical abnormalities. CFS is usually initiated by a major stress, either physical, infectious or emotional.

Much of the dichotomy between body and mind is the result of René Descartes (1596-1650) ideas. Descartes wrote *De homine* in 1633. Because of its political implications, it was not published until after his death. He reasoned that external stimuli affects peripheral nerves which could lead to reflex changes within the nervous system. According to Descartes, the rational soul is an entity distinct from the body and makes contact with the body through the pineal gland. The soul might or might not be aware of the activity inside the brain, but when awareness occurs as a result of conscious sensation, the body affects the mind, which may then perform a voluntary act. He thought of the mind as pure thought and is generally credited with the intense and virtually complete separation of body and mind that followed in medicine and science to the current day.

When we consider the development of the body, starting with two cells that meet and began to divide, it is obvious that everything in the entire body, including the brain and the heart, came from those two cells. The earliest major differentiation is the development of the brain and spinal cord. The surface of this little ball of cells invaginates, creating a rudimentary nervous system. Then, gradually, the other organs begin to differentiate within the body as the fetus develops.

Waking consciousness is physically activated through a small area in the midbrain. The cerebral cortex acts as a giant computer, integrating the many functions of the brain, and allowing the interplay between body, mind and emotion. We know that if the entire right cerebral hemisphere is removed in a child before the age of six, only minimal problems with coordination in the left side of the body result. If the entire left cerebral cortex is removed, the same thing happens, although speech may be lost for some months. Language is generally totally recovered, although the right side will continue to have a very slight problem with coordination.

The cerebral cortex is divided into four major lobes: frontal, temporal, parietal and occipital. The frontal lobes have primarily to do with personality; temporal lobes primarily with memory, with music associated with the right temporal lobe. The parietal lobes are associated with motor function and sensation. In almost 99 percent of people, speech is located in a small area at the junction of the parietal and temporal lobe called Broca's area. In a small percentage of left-handed people, speech is located in the same area on the right side. Occipital lobes have to do with the integration of vision. The cerebellum lies behind the major cortices, and governs fine coordination.

Deep within the brain there are many other groups of cells and areas that have to do with emotions. The hypothalamus is the central control area for the entire maintenance of virtually all bodily functions. Moving further back, to the base of the brain, we have pathways that connect the brain down to the spinal cord and ultimately to the body itself, the central nervous system. There are twelve cranial nerves that control various functions from smell to hearing to taste to chewing—even movement of the neck and shoulders. The spinal cord has both sensory and motor nerves, that allow sensory input from the body and motor activity. Motor activity may be initiated by conscious actions, though built-in reflexes allow quick withdrawal from painful stimuli. In addition, from the second thoracic vertebra down to the lumbar segment of the spinal cord, another series of nerves called the autonomic nervous system lies adjacent to the spine. This includes the sympathetic nervous system, which is responsible for fight or flight, and the parasympathetic, which is responsible for the vegetative or homeostatic digestive system. The autonomic nervous system is particularly associated with hypothalamic control.

Walter Penfield, M.D., a neurosurgeon from Montreal's McGill University, was one of the first researchers to demonstrate that stimulation of various areas of the brain could produce specific actions, from movement to sensation. When the stimulus takes place in the temporal lobes, memories—some long-forgotten—can be evoked.[3]

In the last fifty years, with the evolving use of computers, the brain has often been referred to as the ultimate computer. But Roger Penrose, Ph.D., eminent physicist and mathematician, argues in *The Emperor's New Mind* (1989) that there are many facets of human thinking that can never be emulated by a machine. Penrose argues that quantum mechanics is incomplete and there are laws much deeper than quantum mechanics that are essential for the operation of the mind. He clearly believes that the human mind is much more than a collection of wires and switches. Ultimately, Penrose argues that computation cannot evoke pleasure or pain, cannot perceive poetry or beauty, cannot hope or love or despair, and cannot develop a truly autonomous purpose. He considers consciousness too complex to have been accidentally evoked by a sophisticated mental computer.[4]

Perhaps the best discourse on this subject is *Descartes' Error: Emotion, Reason and the Human Brain* by Antonio Damasio, Ph.D.[5] Damasio argues not only that philosophers were wrong to separate brain and body, but that psychology has been in error by separating reason from emotion. Damasio, Chairman of the Department of Neurology at the University of Iowa, states that there is total interdependence between body and mind. In other words, our physical experience to the world is critical to the creation of our sense of self and markedly influences our behavior. Damasio's work began with review of the study of Phineas Gage, a nineteenth century railway worker who suffered severe loss of his left eye and parts of both frontal lobes. His injuries left him unable to make rational judgments about the present and the future. Damasio and his wife have studied many patients with frontal lobe damage who have intact IQ, memory and language, but a lack of feeling and an inability to put current events into context, or make future judgments. Damasio links the anatomical physiological connections of the frontal lobes with the central motor areas and the emotional limbic system that feed forward and backward from both the body surface and internal organs.

There is a little switch in the midbrain that can apparently turn waking consciousness on or off. On two occasions after WWII, British leader Winston Churchill suffered a stroke of a small branch of the basilar artery. He lay in a coma for some time. On both occasions, he recovered virtually complete neurological function and consciousness and actually served as Prime Minister again after these episodes.

In the last two decades, the new science of psycho-neuroimmunology has given us great insight into the interaction of body and mind. It has demonstrated that every thought evokes a neurochemical. Every known neurochemical created in the brain is also produced in various white blood cells, in the intestines, and other parts of the body. The work of researchers at the HeartMath Institute has also demonstrated essentially that the heart has a "mind" of its own. The body has memory, as shown by heart transplant patients who often have a change of personality and emotions. The body appears to store information holographically.

Our perceptions of the world are highly colored by our beliefs. One of the surprises of modern research has been the discovery that there are about ten times the number of bundles of neurons carrying information *back from* the parts of the brain that process sensory information than there are carrying information *to* that portion. If the brain is convinced of something, its "top down" directives can overrule the data flowing "bottom-up" from the 10 percent of neural bundles carrying information up from the senses.

The brain changes state dramatically depending on how we perceive information. New studies of the brain imaging scans of subjects under hypnosis shows that their brains can be induced to "see" colors where, in reality, they are none. They look at common English words, and perceive them to be meaningless.[6] Referring to this new data, Michael Posner, Ph.D. an emeritus professor of neuroscience at the University of Oregon, says, "The idea that perceptions can be manipulated by expectations fundamental to the study of cognition. But now we're really getting at the mechanisms."[7] In research results that appeared in the *Proceedings of the National Academy of Sciences* in June 2005, and reported in a research summary in the *New York Times,* Dr. Amir Raz reported that the perceptions residing in the brain "'overrode brain circuits devoted to reading and detecting conflict.' A number of other studies of brain imaging point to similar top-down brain mechanisms.... Top-down processes override sensory, or bottom-up information, said Dr. Stephen M. Kosslyn, a neuroscientist at Harvard. People think that sights, sounds and touch from the outside world constitute reality. But the brain constructs what it perceives based on past experience, Kosslyn said." Eighteenth-century American wit Mark Twain wrote, "You cannot depend on your eyes when your imagination is out of focus."[8]

In an elegant set of experiments showing how the brain processes information it receives from the senses, Yale University researchers Anna Roe and her colleagues found that perceptions played a critical role in brain function. She says that, "What is surprising about this paper is we found the cortical map reflects our perceptions, not the physical body," adding that, "The brain is reflecting what we are feeling, even if that's not what really happened." An article in *Science* summarizing her research quotes Mriganka Sur, head of the Massachusetts Institute of Technology Department of Brain and Cognitive Sciences, as saying, "This is a fascinating study that cleverly uses a tactile illusion to demonstrate that the brain's representations of the world, and of sensory stimuli that impinge on us, are shaped by the brain's circuitry. In short, our perceptions have a great deal to do with the way our brains are wired." Roe sums it up as follows:

"We think we know what's out there in the physical world, but it's all interpreted by our brains. Everything we sense is an illusion to a degree."[9]

Since our experience of the outer world is conditioned by our beliefs and expectations, and ten times the amount of neural processing is devoted to sending signals top-down, it makes sense for us to line up those beliefs and expectations with our soul's intentions. Our central nervous system then provides a conduit for expression of our soul's perceptions and missions to the environment. This includes communicating the blueprints for health to every cell in our bodies.

We believe that the soul expresses, learns and evolves through the experiences of the body and its most complex physical component, the brain. We see the brain as the place where major coordination of mind, emotions, and perceptions takes place, where consciousness is harbored, and where intention is formed. Body, mind and emotions are all part of the physical expression called life, ultimately coordinated by the soul. They function in perfect harmony while they serve as conduits of the soul. But when cut off from the soul, even the most brilliant brain loses its pacing with the rhythm of the universe. Soul medicine seeks to synchronize the brain with the energy harmonics of soul consciousness.

SECTION IV

Energy, Electricity and Therapy

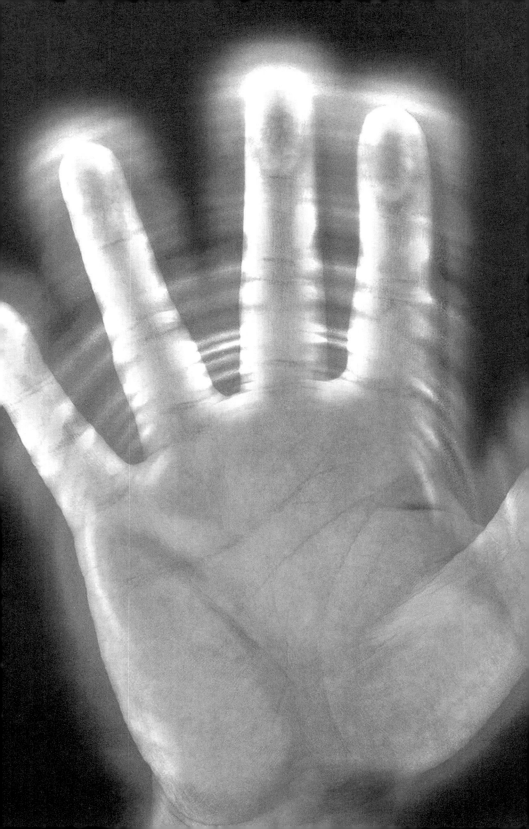

13

The Bodymind Electric

I s it possible that electromagnetic therapy and sacred healing affect the same pathways? Researcher James Oschman hypothesizes that, "any healing that can be accomplished using an electronic device also can be accomplished by a human being."[1] At the University of Colorado Health Sciences Center, research by Dr. John Zimmerman is demonstrating that "the signal practitioners project from their hands correspond in strength and frequency to those produced by various clinical devices that are being developed to stimulate the repair of various kinds of tissues."[2] There are some remarkable parallels between electromagnetic therapies and the work of healers. For much of its history, the study of electricity and magnetism has been closely linked with its applications to wellness. How did the study of electromagnetic energy for health originate?

In 1600, William Gilbert, in his book *De Magnete,* first introduced the concept of electricity and magnetism. He established the difference between electricity (he originated the word) and magnetism, and introduced the concept of magnetic fields. Throughout the seventeenth century, however, such scientists as Descartes and William Harvey insisted that another energy source, an "animating force" or "vital spirit," was necessary to the mechanical physics of the body.

Von Guericke invented the first device for generating electricity in 1660. Newton theorized that Descartes's vital principle, or animating force, was an "all pervading ether" that not only filled the universe but also flowed through nerves in the human body to produce the functions we call life.

Early in the eighteenth century, physicist Stephen Gray discovered that some materials were conductors of electricity. We know today that copper is an excellent conductor, whereas wood or glass shield or prevent conduction. Shortly thereafter, Stephen Hales theorized that nerves might function by conducting electrical powers. However, proof of electrical transmission within the body was not conclusive until 1786, when physiologist Luigi Galvani and his associates discovered that static electricity could travel from outside the body through a nerve inside the body to make a muscle contract. Thus, Galvani decided that "animal electricity" was the long theorized "vital force."

By the mid-1700s, electricity was being artificially generated, stored and transmitted. Quickly, this new discovery became a treatment for a variety of illnesses. The first book concerning the topic was *Electrical Medicine,* published in 1752 by Joharen Schaeffer. A nephew of Galvani, Giovanni Aldini, reported significant improvement and even complete rehabilitation of a schizophrenic with transcranial electrical stimulation.

In 1820, Hans Christian Oersted discovered electromagnetism by demonstrating the effect of electricity upon a compass. In the 1830s, Carlo Matteucci first showed that injured tissues generate an electrical current. Pursuing Matteucci's work, Emil Du Bois-Reymond demonstrated the nerve impulse, the essential mechanism for transfer of information within the nervous system. His colleagues even measured the velocity of a nerve impulse at thirty meters per second. He built an ingenious device to demonstrate the electrical stimulation of nerves. A bowl containing an example of a species of fish that generated occasional electrical discharges was wired to the nerves in a frog's leg. When the fish discharged an electrical pulse, the muscles in the leg contracted. This moved a lever, which rang a bell. Du Bois-Reymond had unknowingly invented biotechnology by becoming the first person to combine biological and mechanical systems in a single device.

Julius Bernstein, in 1868, introduced the concept of bio-electricity, created by the transfer of ions across cell membranes. Today we know that concentrations of potassium and magnesium are higher in cells than outside of them, while extracellular sodium and calcium are higher than intercellular bioelectricity. All these ions carry a positive electrical charge. Their movement, positive across a membrane, generates electricity. Bernstein decided that the impulse was not a current, but a disturbance in the properties of the ions, which ripples along the nerve fiber. The speed of nerve impulses, as measured by Du Bois-Reymond and later scientists, is too slow to be considered a current such as that which runs through a conventional conductor such as copper wire. Du Bois-Reymond's device, and experiments that followed, "served to refute the view held by their teacher, Johannes Müller, that the nerve impulse was an example of a vital function that could never be measured experimentally."[3]

With Bernstein's discovery, the machinists of science quickly rejected electricity in favor of the ion explanation, rooted as it was in conventional chemistry and physics. Chemical changes were much easier to measure than electrical energy. They ignored the fact that the chemical reaction generated electricity! And one hundred and fifty years later, they still have no explanation for where the energy comes from to pump the ions back and forth. The group of scientists of which they were a part founded the German Physical Society in January of 1845. They had no truck with a supposed "vital force." They had "sworn to each other to validate the basic truth that in an organism no other forces have any effect than the common physiochemical ones..." Their work was so influential that it reduced "physiology to applied physics and chemistry, a trend that has dominated physiology and medicine ever since."[4]

Practicing doctors are more pragmatic, and thousands of

nineteenth-century physicians chose to use electricity to treat a variety of problems. That came to a sudden end in 1910 publication of the Flexner Report. Flexner was hired by the American Medical Association to assess medicine in the United States and to assist the AMA in creating an allopathic monopoly. Science and the medical community rejected electrotherapy in favor of physics and chemistry.

Though nonscientific abuses undoubtedly existed in the system, Flexner was a machinist supreme and recommended excommunication of every naturalistic concept of health. Osteopathy, acupuncture and homeopathy were targeted in his zest to expunge "unscientific" practices. Unfortunately, Flexner's report threw out the baby with the bath water; it was accepted as if law.

More than half of all U.S. medical schools and hospitals did not survive Flexner's attack. Homeopathy and acupuncture were relegated to a marginal existence. Osteopathy barely survived the censorship, until the mid-1960s. The American Medical Association fought pitched legal battles to suppress chiropractic.

Since 1910 and the Flexner Report, most aspects of life have improved by way of advances in electric technology and electrification of the world. Few of us would opt to give up electric lighting, cooking appliances, radio, TV, computers, cellphones and the rest of our gadgets. Our enthusiasm for electronics has not translated into a similar flowering of research; the benefits of electrotherapy are still largely unstudied, as well as the negative side effects of artificially generated electromagnetism in our environment.

The medical-scientific black hole created by the Flexner Report resulted in the overlooking of significant findings in Thomas Edison's lab. He showed the induction of a subjective sensation of flickering light when human volunteers were placed in an alternating on-off magnetic field. That is, a magnetic field turned on and off obviously activated the optic visual system to produce a flicker. Somehow this has to be electricity induced in a human brain or eye by magnetism.

Once chemistry became the accepted method by which cells functioned, biochemistry and chemical drugs became the primary foundation of modern medicine. Numerous important electromagnetic experiments were ignored. Among the milestones are these:

- In 1902, a French physician named Leduc reported narcotizing animals with 35 volts of alternating current at 110 cycles per second (Hertz or Hz).

- In 1924, Einthoven won the Nobel Prize for the discovery of the electromagnetic field of the heart. At this time, this required the use of the most sensitive galvanometer available; later instruments permitted the discovery of progressively weaker and subtler fields.

- In 1929, Hans Berger discovered the electroencephalogram, electrical rhythm of the brain. Berger postulated a "bioelectric field." Discovered in 1929, the electrocardiogram (EKG or ECG) has been invaluable in the diagnosis of cardiac disease. Later, the electromyogram (EMG) and nerve conduction testing became essential diagnostic tests for neurology.

- Cerletti in 1938 introduced electroshock therapy for schizophrenia and later depression.

- In the 1940s, physiologists Hodgkin, Huxley and Eccles demonstrated through intracellular nerve cell recordings the generation of electrical discharges by the sodium-potassium exchange.

- Alberg Szent-Gyorgi, the Nobel laureate who discovered the biologic oxidation mechanism of vitamin C, said "Some basic fact about life is still missing." His concept that solid-state electronic processes were generated by biologic molecules reawakened interest in electrobiology.

- A number of investigators demonstrated major influence of DC current on neuronal behavior and a variety of influences

199

of electricity upon brain function, mood, personality and sleep.

- In 1976, Nias demonstrated in double-blind studies the benefits of electrosleep, which had already been used in the USSR for more than twenty-five years. Electrosleep is one of the great unused electrotherapeutic discoveries of this century.

- Eventually the solid-state electronic activity of the neuron system was proven by Ishiko and Lowenstein's demonstration of potential changes induced by raising temperatures without action potential effects in nerve fibers. These and similar DC changes in the eye cannot be explained on the basis of ion exchanges. And indeed, Libet and Gerard had reported in the 1940s electrical brain current of a non-ionic nature, what today would be called "displacement current." Most brain activity is created by intracellular-to-extracellular (and vice versa) movement of sodium, potassium, calcium, and magnesium ions. Electricity and chemistry are inseparable in living organisms.

- In the 1960s Dr. Robert Becker, an orthopedist, and his coworkers demonstrated that currents of only 30 microamps could induce loss of consciousness and general anesthesia in salamanders. They found that an electromagnetic field at strengths of 3000 gauss oriented 90 degrees in a fronto-occipital vector produced similar results. Later experiments demonstrated a magnetic field around the head, with eventual development of a magnetoencephalogram, the magnetic field of the brain, as contrasted with the electrical.

Concomitantly, Becker resurrected early 1900s experiments using electrical current to assist in regenerating tissue regrowth of limbs or tails in salamanders and even of the forearm. But he was not successful in regenerating the paws of cats. His work later led to the development of electrical current that improves healing of fractures of various bones. Becker believed that intrinsic electromagnetic energy inherent in the nervous system of the body is therefore the factor that exerts the major controlling influence over growth processes in general. Indeed, Becker believed electromagnetic property to be intrinsic in all living tissues. Yet the clinical application of his work to healing fractured bones, and the development of the EKG, MRI and EEG, remain some of the very few examples of the use of electromagnetism in healing; most of this area has been a neglected backwater of research for a century.

The Piezoelectronic Connection

Piezoelectric means the ability to convert pressure into electricity. The piezoelectronic property of bone was established in 1954. The piezoelectric mechanism produces an electrical stimulus evoked by mechanical stress or pressure. Becker established the piezoelectrical properties of even collagen, the universal "glue" substance of the body. Dentin, tendon, aorta, trachea, bone, intestines, elastin and nucleic acids are all normal human anatomical transducers of piezoelectro-energy. We are all living piezoelectric generators!

Carrying this correlation of living tissue to electrical phenomena further, others have demonstrated the electromagnetic foundation for activity in the sciatic nerves of frogs, in the growth of bacteria, in the production of carbon dioxide by yeast, in the division of sea urchin eggs, and in cholates, normal bile salts.

Pressure on a tissue, such as occurs during massage, acupressure, or meridian-based therapies, creates a piezoelectric charge. This charge propagates into surrounding tissues. This ripple effect may also have characteristics of a soliton wave. A soliton is a solitary wave that travels at over ten times the speed of the neural signaling network, and was first discovered as the method by which energy is transferred along protein molecules.[5] These very fast signaling mechanisms explain many human abilities that occur at speeds too fast for the neural network: "For example, research has shown that it is impossible to hit a baseball. There is not enough time between the instant a pitcher releases a baseball and the moment it crosses the plate for a hitter to spot it, react to it and swing the bat across the plate to meet it."[6]

The piezoelectric signals created by cells are part of the means by which they communicate with the whole. Becker's work with living systems eventually led him to study the association between externally generated electromagnetic fields and the normal bioelectromagnetics of life itself. Electromagnetic energy activates the piezoelectric property of tissue to emit phonons, which are sound waves with a wavelength low enough to resonate with cell membranes. Thus, electromagnetism activates many of the chemical and physical processes of life. The speed of these phenomena also explains how so many of the physical signaling appears to occur so much faster than can be explained by chemical changes in neural networks.[7]

Indeed it is this bioelectromagnetic aspect that is largely responsible for known and unknown biological cycles or clocks, best known as the circadian or diurnal rhythm (variations during night and day or the twenty-four-hour variations).

In 1954, Frank Brown, a scientist at Northwestern University, demonstrated that oysters that were moved from New Hampshire to Illinois changed the opening and closing of their shells to coincide with the tides at the new location, as if Illinois were a seacoast. Similarly, the night-day timing of many neurochemicals, such as blood levels of cortisol in human beings, change when they are transported great distances longitudinally.

In general, this change is accomplished at a rate of about one hour per day. Thus, a trip from New York to Australia requires at least seven days for a person to accommodate biologically to the new time zone. One of the most critical changes is an individual's production of melatonin, which is essential for good sleep. Jet lag is an example of electromagnetic distortion. Artificially changing one's natural electromagnetic fields by rapidly moving great distances is a twentieth-century development.

During the last thirty years, extensive work has demonstrated that natural electromagnetic phenomena are involved in the migrations of birds, fish and even honeybees. Some bacteria even orient themselves to the earth's magnetic field, apparently because they contain microcrystals of magnetite (the smallest known unit of magnetism). Only recently have similar crystals been found in the human brain. Preliminary research indicates that humans appear to have some electromagnetic tracking sense, which is disrupted when magnets with strengths ranging from 140 to 300 gauss are applied to their heads. Eels tested in the United States are affected by DC electrical fields of 0.67 microvolts/cm and currents of 0.00167 microamps/cm² —truly subtle influences.[8] Becker had calculated that tiny currents would be effective in stimulating cell regrowth, on the order of a billionth of an ampere. He assumed that larger current would be more effective, but when he tested this hypothesis, he found it incorrect. The smaller currents were the most effective, and they correspond to the strength of the human energy field,[9] as surmised by James Oschman, John Zimmerman, and others.

The Influence of Electromagnetic Fields

Central to understanding bioelectromagnetism is the 7 to 10 Hz (cycles per second) frequency that is the dominant rhythm of the Earth and a common frequency component of the EEG readings of all higher animals and humans.

Applied electromagnetic energy can elicit, control or trigger biological changes. Becker emphasized that electromagnetic fields can be stressors. Adrenal production of cortisol, an adrenal hormone essential to life, is significantly altered by pulsed electromagnetic energy. The degree of effect depends on a field's strength and frequency, the duration of exposure (continuous versus intermittent) and even the predisposition of the person being tested.

Electromagnetic waves from television, radio, microwaves, radar, cell phones and satellites bombard us today. These human-made, artificial EMFs overwhelmingly dominate the earth's normal electromagnetic environment—that produced by the sun. Solar influence ensures that almost all areas of the world have electric fields of 0.10/m or greater, and magnetic ones of 100 microgauss or more.

The electromagnetism from human sources ensures that the average exposure of today's humans may be eight to ten times these fields. In the former Soviet Union, "safe" exposure was felt to be below 1 microwatt/cm². We will not know the ultimate epidemiologic health effects of such massive changes in environmental EMFs for many years.

When people are removed from the normal 10 Hz background fields by placing them in specially shielded rooms, their EEGs, mood, and diurnal (day-night) neurochemistry change. The thyroid, pancreas and adrenal glands are all affected by EMFs.

Similarly, cumulative external electromagnetic influences can affect mood, sleep, health and even EEC readings. We now know that electric blankets are extremely dangerous to the fetus in pregnant women, with marked increases in miscarriage and malformations. In patients who are stressed beyond healthy coping ability and have chronic depression, the EEG shows significant asymmetry, most often including

- Excess activity in the right frontal lobe;

- Inability to follow flickering light frequency;

- Excess speeding up or slowing down of EEG signals under the influence of flickering lights;

- Abnormal EEG activity even with an electric clock near the head.

Such individuals sometimes become so sensitive that radio waves may be disturbing to their cognitive congruence.

In Germany, Rutgerin has performed complex experiments on humans in underground, electromagnetically shielded rooms. He has demonstrated that 10 Hz electrical fields assist humans in returning to normal diurnal patterns when they have been destabilized and desynchronized by staying in such shielded rooms.

EEG changes, and alterations to the diurnal rhythms of humans, have been induced by a change of magnetism, applied for only one to three minutes, at 200 to 1,000 gauss, as well as EMFs of 3 to 50 Hz. (The magnetic field of the earth is only 1/2 gauss.) Pulsed EMFs have also been reported to evoke changes in neuronal firing behavior, as well as to affect individual responses to drugs. The threshold for nerve action is lowered and sensitivity to drugs increased. Such effects may occur at levels of EMFs as low as 30 microwatts/cm². In samples of human tissue cultured in labs, minute amounts of electromagnetic energy can affect brain tissue production of norepinephrine. An electric light uses far greater amounts of energy: 120 volts of current, and 40-150 watts of energy.

Biological effects can occur at electromagnetic levels well below those of thermal energy. Animals exposed to higher levels of energy, such as 200-300 gauss for seventy hours, show major anatomical damage to their brain tissue. Even 60 microwatts/cm² of 3 GHz energy applied for up to six weeks causes brain damage.

EMFs can influence the degree of aggression, avoidance patterns, and sleep patterns of animals. Pulsed magnetic fields change humans' reaction times. Even 1 gauss of 60 Hz can alter human concentration. Extremely low EMFs of just .00001 volts can alter EEGs. The multinational pharmaceutical company Ciba-Giegy received a patent for genetic modifications they made to fish eggs, and plants, using only electrical fields. "They were able to grow trout having distinctive hooked jaws that had been extinct for 150 years."[10]

In nonendocrine tissues, the rhythm of the heart can be easily altered by EMFs. And, at extremely low levels, EMFs of 25 to 50 microwatts/cm² can change white blood cells dramatically. Becker concludes, "There is no biological function which can be said to be impervious to non-thermal EMFs—they are a fundamental and pervasive factor in the biology of every living organism."[11]

Beneficial therapies applying EMFs are increasing. Perhaps the most pervasive use has been cardiac pacing. Millions of lives have been gratifyingly and effectively prolonged with pacemakers. Pain control, through TENS (transcutaneous electrical nerve stimulator) units, or electroacupuncture, is also at the forefront of bioelectromagnetic therapy.

Electrodermal screening is a technology developed in West Germany just after WWII. It was originated by biophysicist Dr. Reinhard Voll, who discovered a means of measuring the electrical characteristics of acupuncture points. His experiments used a skin galvanometer to measure electrical differentials when a subject was exposed to various potential toxins and allergens. He later extended his tests to determine what remedies might be most effective in correcting these conditions. There are some 100,000 electrodermal screening units in use worldwide, but very few in the United States; the unit's operating principles using quantum physics and energy medicine have prevented it from gaining wide acceptance.[12] Yet there are many accounts of the detection of diseases, allergies and toxic states using EDS machines—detection before these conditions reach the threshold at which they can be medically chronicled.[13]

Magnetic Therapy

In her book *Energy Medicine,* Donna Eden summarizes studies by the International Council of Magnetic Therapists that suggest that "magnets have produced improvements in a wide range of medical conditions, including tendonitis, blood circulation, diabetic neuropathy, bone cysts, hypertension, optic nerve atrophy, facial paralysis, and fracture healing."[14]

Dr. Dean Bonlie graduated with honors from Loma Linda School of Dentistry. He has devised a magnetic sleep pad which is quite remarkable. The earth's magnetic field just 4,000 years ago is estimated by geoscientists to have been 2.5 gauss. Today it is only 0.5 gauss. Cleopatra is reported to have worn a lodestone (a magnetic stone) on her forehead to retard aging. Dr. Bonlie believes that chronic fatigue syndrome and fibromyalgia are diseases of magnetic deficiency. Interestingly, magnesium deficiency is also rampant in these individuals. Magnesium is named for magnetics. Bonlie's work has demonstrated that sleeping on his Magnetico pad decreases red blood cell clumping, markedly improves fibromyalgia, and provides relief in a variety of pain problems, allergies, migraines, hypertension, diabetes, and insomnia. There is increasing evidence that this magnetic therapy improves heart disease and circulation and may be helpful in multiple sclerosis. Indeed, my (Norm Shealy) blood pressure goes from 120/80 to 94/60 when I lie on the Magnetico mattress pad. And the electroencephalogram in everyone we have tested immediately shifts into the deepest states of relaxation we have seen at our clinic.[15]

The Secret of Life

Throughout history, philosophers and mystics have pondered about the energy of life itself. In every culture, except that of modern scientific monotheism, life is considered sacred, the physical manifestation of spiritual energy emanating from a divine source. Though the majority of us share common beliefs, science has ignored or suppressed interest in the nature of life itself since the days of Rene Descartes' infamous statement, "I think; therefore I am."

The concept of thinking itself is poorly understood by scientists, religious leaders and laypersons because it defies scientific explanation. *The Random House College Dictionary* defines thinking as "1. rational; reasoning; 2. thoughtful; reflective; studious." In an attempt to make humans the ultimate creation, many scientists have insisted that animals don't think, plan, play or have emotions. This seems hard to believe when you associate with animals and watch their behavior! Ignorance, as Dr. Edward Bach (1886-1936) defined it, is simply the failure to accept truth.

Energy is the basic framework of the universe, down to individual atoms. Life energy is simply one aspect of consciousness. The study of electromagnetism is exciting because with the right experimental designs, it allows us to detect the influence of unseen energies, soul presence, and consciousness. Soul medicine is introducing the medical establishment to a new model of health, one that understands that energy and consciousness play a vital part in healing. The body's electromagnetic field is a means through with biochemistry and physical anatomy interact with unseen energies.

The Electromagnetic Framework of Life

China, the oldest continuous civilization, considers life to be a result of *chi* or *qi*. Chi is believed to come from the universe and flow through the body in channels or meridians. A German scientist, Wilhelm Reich (1897-1957), one of the few psychiatrists to consider life energy and study it scientifically, referred to life energy as *orgone*.

A Russian engineer, Georges Lakhovsky (1869-1942), published his book *The Secret of Life* more than seventy-five years ago in which he declared the vibratory frequency of DNA to be 50-plus billion cycles per second, or Gigahertz. Modern Ukrainian quantum physicists have taken Lakhovsky's concepts much further and refer to it as the study of Giga-energy. They report that human DNA vibrates at 52 to 78 Gigahertz (billions of cycles per second); that of animals at 47 Gigahertz; and that of plants at 42 Gigahertz. They believe that each individual resonates most significantly at a unique, eigen or individual frequency. Thus, there could be 27 billion specific frequencies, from 52 billion cycles per second up to 78 billion cycles per second.

Furthermore, these physicists believe each human organ, because of its anatomic structure, projects its vector, or energy, along a specific pathway for that organ, the acupuncture meridian for that organ. This subtle Giga-energy—at a mere *one-billionth* of a watt per cm^2—may be the electromagnetic support system for chi. Researcher James Oschman, in a brilliant synthesis of the field of energy healing, declares that, "living systems are far more sensitive to the energetic environment than we realized. ...One reason is that cells contain molecular amplifiers and signal processors that are far more sophisticated than anything physicists or electronic engineers have dared dream of." A British researcher, Mae-Wan Ho, points out that the crystalline structure of cells within tissues, and of the arrangement of tissues within organs, has important consequences, as the structure resonates harmonically: "When the coherence builds to a certain level...the organism behaves as a single crystal. ...A threshold is reached where all the atoms oscillate together in phase and send out a giant light track that is a million times stronger than that emitted by individual atoms."[16]

Chi may be susceptible to measurement by studying levels of the most common human hormone, DHEA (dehydroepiandrosterone). DHEA declines after age thirty in most people. DHEA manifests from cholesterol, and cholesterol increases in many persons after age thirty. Might a correlation exist between DHEA and cholesterol, perhaps due to an acquired enzyme deficiency? In a preliminary study, seven men were given supplemental progesterone. Their DHEA levels rose between 30 percent and 100 percent, with an average increase of 60 percent. DHEA levels decline with every known illness. Cumulative stress may also produce a decline in DHEA, since it may be the chemical battery reflecting the level in our life energy reservoirs.[17]

Emotional Cures Via Orgasmic Bioelectrical Release

The third most influential psychiatrist in history, Wilhelm Reich, set out to answer whether a sexual orgasm is an essentially mechanical process. Freud considered orgasm to be simply a "mechanical" release. This limited mechanistic view led psychiatrists to conclude it was not natural for women to experience orgasm since they had no mechanical release, or ejaculation!

Reich felt that orgastic potency was the key to understanding emotional life in general and psychic disorders or neuroses in particular. Thus Reich assumed that sexual tension and relaxation require a "bioelectrical discharge" during orgasm.

Reich noted that genital friction led to involuntary genital muscle contracture, greater with gentle, slow friction than vigorous, rapid friction. He noticed that people who had a high degree of body armoring required vigorous movement to produce stimulation.

Reich claimed that the basic function of all living matter, namely tension and relaxation, charge and discharge, were part of the natural function of orgasm. Orgastic bioelectric discharge produced pleasure and relaxation. Blockage resulted in tension, anxiety and separation from the partner. Thus he considered orgasm "one of the most important modal points of the body-soul problem."[18]

In orgastic function the first requirement is vegetative excitation and increased blood flow to the genitals, a function of the parasympathetic nervous system. Activation of the sympathetic nervous system leads to the constriction of the arteries, and decreased blood flow to the genitals. Reich noted that the involuntary muscle tension created by genital friction was the same as that created by electrically stimulating muscles. Eventually the friction leads to muscle clonus—involuntary automatic contractions concomitant with orgasm. The mechanical friction and tension builds an electrical charge, which must lead to both mechanical and electrical discharge. He insisted that post-orgasmic relaxation was not mechanical but bioelectric.

Thus he considered the normal, natural process of orgasm to be tension > discharge > relaxation, the centerpiece of his concept of expansion-contraction as the governing principle in life itself. Mechanical tension, he determined, led to an electrical discharge, and electrical discharge led to mechanical relaxation. He felt that this link between mechanics and electricity was also a distinguishable characteristic of living matter.

Reich emphasized that the sympathetic system acts like calcium—it produces tension—whereas the parasympathetic system acts like potassium, leading to relaxation. He further believed that cholesterol is like calcium and lecithin like potassium. Alkalines behave like potassium and acids like calcium.

There is an antithesis between sexuality and anxiety—the parasympathetic leads to peripheral excitation and central relaxation of sexual expansion; the sympathetic leads to peripheral relaxation and central excitation or anxiety.

Electrical discharge in muscles leads to mechanical relaxation. As mechanical muscle tension builds, the piezoelectric effect increases the voltage gradient. At some critical gradient electric overload occurs, leading to that electrical discharge.

Sexual arousal is an electrical charging of the erogenous surfaces. Orgasm is a discharge of the potential accumulated during stimulation-activation. Reich concluded that orgasm is a basic manifestation of living substance, and the tension-charge formula cannot be applied to nonliving nature.

Skin response to emotions changes electrical potential and resistance, the electrical function of sexual zones being different from that of the rest of the skin. Sexual skin (genitals, tongue, lips, nipples, ears) have other much higher or lower potential than nonsexual skin. "Muscular motor activity in general and rhythmic friction, the rubbing together of pleasurably excitable body surfaces, are the fundamental biological phenomena of sexuality."[19] Friction without pleasure does not increase potential. Friction with pleasure does. In anxiety or annoyance, surface potential decreases.

Reich believed that the vegetative muscle system is the generator of bioelectrical energy in the human body. Since sexually responsive skin is the only skin that responds with marked increase in potential, he concluded that sexual activity is the bioenergetic productive process itself.

Obviously, all muscle tension is part of the total bioelectrical energy system. A half-century ago, Yale University professor Harold Saxton Burr named it the "electro-dynamic field." Based on over twenty years of experiments, he argued that illnesses, both psychological and physical, show up in the energy field long before they manifest as concrete pathologies. Conversely, the physical disease could be treated by restoring balance to the energy system.[20] The degenerative diseases may also be helped by the general improvement of a patient's energy systems through alternative medicine. Degenerative diseases may be the result of energy blockages and the loss of cooperation among the subtle energy systems of the whole network of life. These conditions can be improved only by energy medicine. Oschman calls this field the *living matrix*. Here's how he summarizes the properties of the components of the living matrix. Notice that all but one of them are electromagnetic characteristics:

1. **Semiconduction.** All of the components are semiconductors. This means they can both conduct and process vibrational information, much like an integrated circuit or microprocessor in a computer. They also convert energy from one form to another.

2. **Piezoelectricity**. All of the components are piezoelectric. This means that waves of mechanical vibration moving through the living matrix produce electrical vields and vice versa...

3. **Crystallinity**. Much of the living matrix consists of molecules that are regularly arrayed in crystal-like lattices. This includes lipids in cell membranes, collagen molecules of connective tissue, actin and myosin molecules of muscle, and components of the cytoskeleton.

4. **Coherency**. The highly regular structures just mentioned produce giant coherent or laser-like oscillations that move rapidly throughout the living matrix and that also are radiated into the environment.

5. **Hydration**. Water is a dynamic component of the living matrix. On average, each matrix protein has 15,000 water molecules associated with it....

6. **Continuity**: As we have seen, the properties just listed are not localized but are spread throughout the organism. Although we may distinguish individual organs, tissues, cells, and molecules, the living matrix is a continuous and unbroken whole.[21]

In its component parts, and in its aggregate whole, our bodies, souls, minds and emotional realms are interrelated energy systems. Energetic treatment of one part of this living matrix always affects the whole. This explains otherwise-mysterious effects, such as why massage stimulates memory. Massage therapists have long noticed that manipulation of certain muscles produces emotional experiences in their clients. A client may spontaneously recall a long-forgotten childhood wounding experience when a certain muscle is touched, along with all the emotions associated with the event. Wilhelm Reich was the first to explain in detail that accumulations of memories in the tissue could lead to rigid muscles, or "body armoring." Release of the tension held in the organ can result in a release of the emotion surrounding the event, especially when this phenomenon is used by a skilled therapist.

Massage and other forms of bodywork also stimulate the body's connective tissue. All the body's systems are contained within a protective sheath of connective tissue. Connective tissue is a liquid crystalline semiconductor. Piezoelectric signals from the cells can travel throughout the body in this medium. Oschman adds, "If the parts of the organism are cooperative and coordinated in their functioning and every cells knows what every other cell is doing, it is due to the continuity and signaling properties of the connective tissue."[22] Connective tissue is a vital component in the harmonious coordination of the body's energy fields

Acupuncture: An Ancient EMT Technique

Acupuncture is the oldest known form of energetic medicine. There is more valid scientific proof of its effectiveness than any other nonconventional therapy; over one thousand studies testify to its effectiveness in treating a wide range of complaints. Acupuncture may be considered the foundation for an understanding of electromagnetic principles in healing.

Although acupuncture has flourished in China for 4,000 years, modern Western medicine rejected it until recently. Interestingly, Sir William Osier considered acupuncture the "treatment of preference" in lumbago (low back pain) in 1912. We have used it for decades to treat pain and many other symptoms.

213

Dr. Robert Becker, exploring the body's semiconductive capabilities, demonstrated that the tissues around nerves were such semiconductors. He postulated that acupuncture points were areas of amplifier boosters built along transmission cables to propagate electrical signals. Many other investigators have shown that acupuncture points have lower electric resistance than nonacupuncture points. Pomeranz showed that acupunctured points had injury current as high as 10 microamps and this current's injury lasts several days. Dr. William Tiller, Stanford University professor of materials science, postulates that there is a magnetic field above acupuncture channels that creates a battery-like effect at acupuncture points with increased electrical conductivity. This battery would then represent part of a complex electrical system emanating from individual organs.

Ukrainian nuclear physicists postulate such a vector system. For instance, heart DNA cells resonate at 52 to 78 billion cycles per second and radiate a vector along specific pathways (meridians) to the tips of the fingers or toes, with a resonating circuit back to the organ. Dr. Hans Popp, a German scientist, believes there are many charged oscillators in the body that send out a variety of electromagnetic waves, some of which are emitted from the body. Dr. Nordstrom, a Swedish physician, postulates that living electrical circuits travel in the fascial tissue around blood vessels, as well as interconnecting with the electrical circuits of nerves. Careful dissection of cadavers by bodywork students has drawn attention to tiny fibers coursing through the connective tissue and fascia of the body, in patterns that closely resemble the ancient Chinese charts showing acupuncture meridians.[23]

Acupuncture Principles

Acupuncture meridians are located near the surface of the body between muscle groups. Acupuncture points lie in the depressions between muscle groups. The points coexist with deeper muscle-nerve points (the actual nerve interface with the muscle) 75 percent of the time.

Acupuncture needles are stainless steel with a contrasting metal handle. This bimetallic effect is one of three mechanisms that make acupuncture an inherent electrical treatment. When two different metals are placed in a salt solution, a current flow is created by the different electrical conductivity of the two metals. Secondly, the tip of the needle in the body is warmer than the handle (perhaps 25°F or greater), creating an electrical gradient. The spiral handle is a radiator, proving a larger surface area than the tip. Electrons transfer from one metal to the next as needle temperature varies and the handle oxidizes.

The tip of the needle becomes positive relative to the handle. If the handle is heated or manually twirled, the tip becomes negative, providing additional electrical flow. It takes sixty to ninety minutes for such flow to reach equilibrium. Two needles physically separated in the body on two different acupuncture points thus electrically connect by an electron wave from the twirling, heated or electrically stimulated needle to a stable needle not manipulated.

Ancient Chinese did not understand or describe electrical circuits. They talked about a life force circulating in the body's meridians to protect, nourish and animate all life, generating warmth and stimulating all bodily functions and organs. Such a concept is universal. Ancient Greeks called it "pneuma"; eastern Indians "prana"; Paracelsus called it "quintessence"; Galvani labeled it "animal electricity"; Hahnemann, father of homeopathy, referred to it as the "vital force"; and Mesmer "magnetism." Modern medicine uses only the term "vitality" and has little concept of a circuit for this vitality.

Modern studies of acupuncture's benefits include the following, drawn from the many scientific studies showing the effectiveness of acupuncture:

- Greater improvement of osteoarthritis than a much-prescribed drug.[x]

- Improvement in PMS (premenstrual syndrome) with treatment of the sexual circuit (Tchong Mo).[y]

- Restoration of fertility in two-thirds of infertile men through treatment of the Tchong Mo circuit. One man increased his sperm count from 9 to 54 million (a 600 percent increase), which could not be accomplished with any modern medical approach.[26]

- Control of chronic tension headaches in approximately three-quarters of patients.[27]

- Restoration of DHEA levels in two-thirds of individuals.

- Reduction in the chest pain of heart patients who had been unresponsive to conventional drugs.[28]

Chinese divide *qi* into *Wei Qi, Rong Qi,* and *Yuan Qi, Wei Qi,* is produced by digestion and internal organ metabolism. It is said to surround the body like a shield, preventing environmental forces from affecting the inner channels. *Wei Qi* controls sweating, warmth, and the integrity of the skin and superficial fascia.

Rong Qi is the end product of the total vitality received from food and drink, mixed with inhaled air. Rong Qi circulates with blood inside the body as well as in the energy channels that link organs with the surface of the body. Rong Qi is both the result of, and essential to, balanced functioning of the internal organs.

Original energy, *Yuan Qi,* is the genetic, inherited, constitutional energetic component. It is the precursor of all other qi, is not reversible, and is responsible for growth, development, reproduction, transformation and aging. It resides in the kidney and circulates through extra channels that regulate or balance all energy in the body. Since it cannot be replaced, Yuan Qi is greatly respected, as it can be depleted by physical, mental, emotional or sexual exhaustion, or an unwise diet.

The twelve meridians are the principal circuits for energy circulation. They allow qi to move constantly. Acupuncture needles are used to activate the circuits, adding or subtracting energy to balance deficient or excess energy in any organ.

In one sense, the Chinese expressed the essence of electrical "charge" with their concept of yin and yang, negative and positive. Chinese cosmology also includes descriptions of elements. These are wood (flexibility, relatively yang), fire (brilliance, passion, yang), Earth (solidity, balanced yin-yang), metal (structural integrity, relatively yin) and water (fluidity, yin). According to acupuncture's principles:

- Kidney, a yang organ, manages water, osmotic regulation and fluid excretion (a description totally compatible with Western medicine). It also is associated with adrenal and sexual function.

- Heart, a yin organ, not only pumps blood but energetically expresses spirit and creativity, a widespread metaphysical concept.

- Small intestine is responsible for digestion and absorption of food and liquid (as in Western medicine).

- Bladder regulates the elimination of fluid (as in modern medicine) and partially controls the central nervous system, along with the kidney. (The latter is an interesting analogy, since brain function is so remarkably related to cerebrospinal fluid production, absorption and circulation.)

- Liver and gallbladder are "wood" organs. Certainly the liver is the most flexible of all organs.

- Master of the Heart (sympathetic system) and Triple Master (parasympathetic) are "fire organs," and nothing is more synchronous with the fire of the body than the autonomic nervous system, which includes adrenalin, the "fire" chemical for reaction to stress.

- Stomach (Earth) and large intestine (metal) involve all aspects of digestion, just as in modern medicine.

- Spleen (Earth) is concerned with blood (as in modern medicine) and includes pancreatic function in Chinese energetics.

- Lung (metal) includes respiration.

- Skin is considered an organ of respiration, which, when we consider sweating, is not too far-fetched in modern Western terms.

Acupuncture is an ancient technique for activation of the electromagnetic system. Insertion of a metal needle into a chemical reservoir, the body, generates a flow of electricity. "Reports from Japan and China have shown that the projected qi includes a strong magnetic component that can be detected with a simple magnetometer."[29] Beyond that, the effects of acupuncture may be a subtle form of sacred healing.

Other forms of meridian-based therapies are now being studied. These use the same meridian pathways, but do not use needles. Usually they involve constant pressure, like Shiatsu massage, tapping with a fingertip (EFT, or Emotional Freedom Therapy, the technique used by Dr. Robins to treat Michele in Chapter One), or self-pressure (like the Tapas Acupressure Technique or TAT). The mechanism by which these therapies work is probably piezoelectricity; tapping on tissues generates an electric current. Tapping on meridians produces results, whereas studies in which a control group uses random or sham tapping shows that this non-meridian tapping is not as effective.

One study of EFT, published in the *Journal of Clinical Psychology* in 2003, examined patients who had severe clinical phobias. These patients had disabling fears of small animals such as bats, snakes, spiders and rats. Having a clinical phobia doesn't mean you dislike something. These patients had severe reactions, which the researchers measured in four ways: a pulse rate test, a written questionnaire, a subjective stress test, and an objective stress test consisting of how many steps toward the animal the subject could take.

They were then given a half hour explanation of EFT that included one brief EFT treatment. EFT treatments usually take under two minutes.

Patients were then re-tested, and showed a significant

improvement in every single measure of stress.[30] One woman was severely phobic to mice, and would sleep in her car if she even imagined there was a mouse in the house. She could not enter the room with the mouse during the preliminary examination.

After EFT, she walked into the room containing the mouse, and examined the creature curiously. Her daughter later purchased a rat for her grand-daughter, and in a television interview she was seen holding the rat and remarking that they don't seem like such scary creatures after all. A follow up examination, six months later, found that the reduction in phobic behavior had stuck. These are amazing results from two minutes of meridian therapy! James Oschman, whose summaries of the field of electromagnetic healing elegantly synthesize every important trend, speculates that, "tapping interacts directly with the electronic system within the body that stores traumatic and other memories.... By asking a patient to focus on his or her emotional discomfort while tapping on the points, the therapist is directly interacting with the flows of energy and information related to the original emotional state or phobia."[31]

Acupressure, acupuncture, meridian-based therapies, electrical activation of energetic circuits, and other methods of enhancing the body's electromagnetic potential for healing are quick, cheap, mostly non-invasive, and harmless. They can have effects out of all proportion to their cost and complexity. Making them the first line of treatment could solve virtually all of society's problems with its current medical system—limited access, high cost, low touch, excessive complexity, iatrogenic illness and death—at a single stroke.

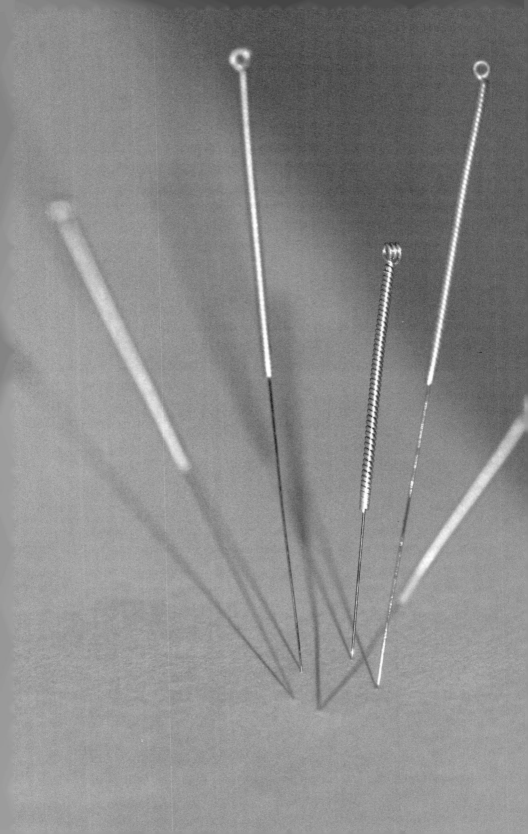

14

Shifting the Pain Paradigm

NORMAN SHEALY, M.D., PH.D.

Electrotherapy has intrigued naturalist physicians for almost 2,000 years. In 46 A.D., Scribonius Largus described how an electric ray was used to treat both headaches and painful gout. In the late nineteenth and early twentieth centuries, electrotherapy peaked in popularity. It was claimed to cure virtually every conceivable symptom or illness. The Bakken Library in Minneapolis has a magnificent collection of devices, some as large as a room, all claiming in their day to cure virtually everything.

The Electreat

Ultimately, only one of the popular devices survived the witch hunt of the Flexner Report: the Electreat, patented in 1919 by C. W. Kent, a naturopath from Peoria, Illinois. The device remained on the market through the 1940s, despite intense attack by the FDA and rejection by the medical profession.

In 1951, my father suffered from a painful facial paralysis called Bell's palsy. Unsuccessfully treated by several physicians, he consulted a chiropractor who prescribed an Electreat. The device provided him with relief from the pain, and full recovery. In 1960, when I had neck and arm pain from a ruptured cervical disc, my father gave me his Electreat. Because of its somewhat clumsy design and my lack of insight into its potential, I barely used it. However, I was impressed by the many claims of its curative power and the machine's peculiar ability to pass an electrical current from one person to another.

Then, a seemingly inconsequential event in 1963 brought the Electreat back into my awareness. Dr. William Collins, a neurosurgeon, left Western Reserve University, where both of us were on the faculty, and moved to Virginia. He had begun studying pain physiology before I arrived at the university. As a joke, I presented him with the Electreat at his going-away party. Together, we laughed at the snake-oil design of its internal electrode and electric comb. In 1965, Pat Wall of MIT introduced his concept of the spinal gate as the physiological mechanism for pain. He demonstrated that the smallest "C" nerve fibers enter the spinal cord with pain information and may there be blocked by input over the largest Beta fibers, which modulate or regulate pain input. This "gate" also can be closed by descending nerve fibers from the brain. I wondered if the Electreat was having its effects by closing that gate. I talked to Dr. Collins, but he had discarded my gift. Yet I discovered that the Electreat was still being produced in Peoria, and I acquired one.

The Dorsal Column Stimulator

In 1965, I introduced the concept of dorsal column stimulation, proving the value of electrical stimulation of the spinal cord's dorsal columns to suppress pain. In April 1967, modern electrotherapy became a reality. I surgically implanted a battery-powered Dorsal Column Stimulator (DCS) into a man who was terminally ill with widespread cancer; and his pain was totally controlled.[1]

Dorsal column stimulation worked well over the next eight years in 75 percent of my patients with chronic pain. Alas, there are risks involved, and the long-term benefits are not significant enough for me to recommend it to most patients with non-cancer pain. Meanwhile, however, nonsurgical tools had been developed that are equally effective in masking chronic pain in at least 85 percent of patients.

The First Modern TENS

I continued to use the Electreat in my practice. At first, I used it to demonstrate the feeling of electrical stimulation to patients who were to receive a DCS. Later, it was used in treatment. From the outset of my electrotherapy study, I was convinced that external surface or skin stimulation would be applicable at least 1,000 times as often as dorsal column stimulation.

As early as 1967, I had encouraged Medtronic design engineers, who had manufactured my Dorsal Column Stimulator, to produce a modern solid-state Electreat. Medtronic refused because they focused on implanted devices; they were the originators of the cardiac pacemaker.

In the early 1970s, Norman Hagfors, a Medtronic design engineer who had worked on my invention, left Medtronic to establish a new company, Stim-Tech, Inc. Before long, he purchased the Electreat Company and moved it to Minnesota. The Electreat continued to be manufactured until 1993. Stim-Tech introduced the first solid-state modern skin stimulator, also called the Stim-Tech. The initial large box (approximately a foot square and four inches thick) emitted a pulsed, square wave. I believed this could not be as effective as the spike-type pulsed waves of the Electreat, and with my urging, Medtronic produced a much smaller device with a spiked wave.

In the three decades since the introduction of this early device, a plethora of TENS (Transcutaneous Electrical Nerve Stimulator) devices flooded the market. However, they never penetrated mass-market consciousness or received a single marketing "push" from a pharmaceutical company. Today, a company called Empi is the major producer of TENS units. Each year, an estimated 100,000 TENS units are sold, with an annual revenue of $100 million. TENS devices relieve approximately 50 percent of chronic pain adequately. Of the 50 million sufferers in the United States, probably only 2 percent have chosen this treatment—although it's the safest pain reliever ever introduced.

I had always insisted that modern TENS machines could not measure up to the effectiveness of an Electreat. Though their pulsations were often somewhat more pleasant, the waves neither penetrated nor traveled nearly as extensively through the body. The whole picture became apparent only in 1994, after I discovered GigaTENS. Now, four decades after my first explorations, I have been able to redesign a device that puts out the frequencies of the old Electreat, but in a modern package, with modern electrodes and controls. The SheLi TENS is the first device I've allowed to use my name. I believe that the energy of the SheLi TENS comes as close as we can get to mobilizing the body's chi with electrotherapy.

Cranial Electrical Stimulation

In 1975, before the FDA placed restrictions on medical devices, Dr. Saul Liss, a medical engineer, introduced his TENS device. Initially called the Pain Suppressor, it was later redesigned and renamed the Liss Body Stimulator and another model was called the Liss Cranial Electrical Stimulator. The machine did not impress me on first try because it emitted only 4 milliamps of current, which generally is lower than sensory perception. When Saul made me a 10 milliamp unit, though, I had to admit it was too strong.

By chance, I touched one of the electrodes to my forehead about 10:30 one night. It evoked a sensation of flickering lights. For the next hour, I experimented with the machine in various positions. No matter where on the cranial vault one or both of the electrodes were placed, I saw a visual flicker. The flicker was there even with one electrode on top of my head and the other on my foot.

I went to bed about 11:30 P.M. and awoke at 2:30 A.M., unable to sleep any longer because of marked increased energy and alertness.

A few months later my associate, Dr. James Kwako, and I both applied this device transcranially at 8:00 A.M. for forty-five minutes. Four hours later my blood serotonin level had increased to five times the upper limit of normal, and Dr. Kwako's had doubled.

Dr. Kwako and I decided to try Saul's device on patients with depression. The first patient, from Florida, had been depressed for sixteen years. Remarkably, an hour of transcranial stimulation completely relieved his depression in just one day. Unfortunately, he insisted on returning home to Florida with no more treatments; within one week, his depression returned.

These two findings—serotonin elevation and the relief of depression—motivated me to study the Liss Body Stimulator further. Serotonin is one of the body's most important neurochemicals, involved in mood regulation, sleep and pain. Serotonin-modulating drugs have been extensively studied for the treatment of depression, as well as for migraine headaches.

I treated seventy-five patients with chronic pain with the Liss machine. Forty percent of them had a serotonin deficiency, while the other 40 percent had excessive serotonin. They received an hour a day of treatment with the Liss device for two weeks, after which their serotonin levels were tested again. Analysis revealed that, in 80 percent of the group, serotonin output was now normal. Their self-reported mood swings had also abated.

I determined that when the Liss unit was used transcranially, it relieved depression in 50 percent of chronically depressed patients who had failed to respond earlier to one or more antidepressant drugs. More recently, we have found that photostimulation, education and vibratory music also relieve depression in 58 percent of chronically depressed patients. But when we combine the two approaches, using a Liss device along with photostimulation, education and vibratory music, a striking 85 percent of patients come out of depression. With no further therapy, 70 percent remain free of depression three to six months later. At this point, we recommend continued use of the Liss Cranial Stimulator, Shealy Series (modified to allow one hour of therapy) once or twice a week after the initial daily treatment program.

The Liss device used transcranially is also remarkably helpful in treating insomnia and in overcoming jet lag. It has enhancing effects on beta endorphin, the natural "feel good" narcotic, as well as upon serotonin. DHEA production is enhanced when the Liss unit is applied to a specific pattern of acupuncture points. There may be a variety of other uses as well.

I believe that every household should have a TENS device. Unfortunately, purchase of a TENS requires a prescription. Most physicians know virtually nothing about the benefits this device can provide. Because no pharmaceutical company sponsors the TENS, it is likely to continue to be underused unless patients insist that their physicians prescribe it.

GigaTENS

In December 1992, Saul Liss and I were invited to visit Kiev, in the Ukraine, to study a device called the MRT (Microwave Resonance Therapy). According to the hosting quantum physicists, they had discovered this approach twelve years earlier. They said they had learned that

- Human DNA resonates at 54 to 78 billion cycles-per-second (gigahertz);

- Animal DNA resonates at 47 gigahertz;

- Plant DNA resonates at 42 gigahertz.

Furthermore, they reported curing 50 percent of narcotic addicts, 92 percent of alcoholics, and more than 80 percent of patients with rheumatoid arthritis when applying 54 to 78 gigahertz at one-billionth of a watt to selected acupuncture points. More than 200,000 patients had been treated with the MRT. Therapy usually lasted a total of thirty minutes per day, five days per week, for two weeks, with remission or a cure occurring for up to two years.

The physicians were treating virtually every illness with MRT, from angina pectoris to diabetes to osteomyelitis (chronic infections of bone). No complications from this therapy were reported.

Liss and I, working with two Ukrainian physicists, redesigned the device to use in clinical situations. We call the device the GigaTENS and have verified this technology's benefits. Striking pain relief is realized in 70 percent of patients with rheumatoid arthritis for whom conventional drug therapy has failed. Pain relief and some neurological improvement are seen in 80 percent of patients with diabetic neuropathy. GigaTENS improves 50 percent of patients with chronic back pain or depression. GigaTENS therapy appears to be one of the most versatile, safe and effective therapies known to date.

Now that the equipment to test giga-frequencies was available, in the summer of 1994, I tested my old favorite, the Electreat. It became clear why I have always preferred the Electreat—it puts out a giga-frequency. Amazingly, C. W. Kent had marketed a prototype of GigaTENS in 1919. Considering the experience of the Ukrainian physicians, perhaps Dr. Kent was right in some of his elaborate claims.

Dr. William Tiller, a Stanford University materials scientist, and I have now created a smaller, much more user-friendly device, the SheLi TENS, which has all the advantages of TENS units, plus the superior benefits of operating at a giga-frequency. At this point, the SheLi TENS is the safest, most effective stimulator available, the best remedy we know for treatment of pain, depression, insomnia, jet lag, migraine, rheumatoid arthritis and diabetic neuropathy. For pain alone, this device is invaluable. Totally safe, it can be used by virtually everyone except patients with cardiac pacemakers, as the device might interfere with the function of the pacemaker.

Much progress is yet to be made, as new types of electromagnetic stimulators and possibly new applications for this type of device, evolve. The Electreat arrived at the start of the twentieth century. After more than eighty years, it still is more useful than some other modern TENS devices. The SheLi TENS and Liss CES are the first known electrotherapy devices that strikingly alter human neurochemistry. These two devices are a foundation for twenty-first-century energy medicine.

Electroacupuncture

When I began dorsal column stimulation in 1967, I inserted needles into the painful areas on patients' bodies and attached electrical stimulators to them. The importance of inserting the needle into the center of pain soon became apparent. This is a rule in classic acupuncture. By the late 1960s, I was calling my technique PENS (Percutaneous Electrical Nerve Stimulation).

Other than having read some literature about it, I had no formal training in acupuncture. In 1973, I went to England to study with Dr. Felix Mann, a British physician who had trained in France and China and translated several ancient acupuncture texts into English. (Mann ordinarily did not use electrical stimulation of acupuncture needles.)

The Chinese knew about my clinic and my work with electrical stimulation, and the first Chinese medical delegation to come to the U.S. after relations with China opened requested a visit me in late 1973. I learned during that visit that the Chinese had begun applying electrical stimulation through acupuncture needles in 1967—the same year I did.

Most Western practitioners now use electrical stimulation for many acupuncture treatments. It has been shown that stimuli at 1 Hz, 1 cycle per second, raises levels of beta endorphin. Higher frequencies, although they may effectively relieve pain, do not raise beta endorphins.

A number of electrical innovations today attempt to capitalize on electroacupuncture. Many do not use needles but just apply focal shocks to acupuncture points. Little scientific study has been done of these techniques or of lasers applied to acupuncture points.

Electromagnetic Characteristics of Healing

I evaluated the effects of Ostad Parvarandeh's remote healing treatments on patients using EEGs and EKGs of their heart and brain rhythms.

The first group was composed of thirty patients. Ostad was asked to apply healing for about two minutes, after a long control period to establish normal EEG activity. The patient had no knowledge of when healing would be applied, or for how long. Ostad sat in separate room about one hundred feet away. He was given a Polaroid photograph of the patient. We measured the exact time at which Ostad began his healing transmission, and correlated it with the output received by the EEG technician.

The EEG records are reproduced in an appendix to this book. The results are quite striking. They show that, at the exact moment at which Ostad began his treatment, 84 percent had an immediate and often dramatic decrease in alpha wave activity.

Another test, with thirty-two patients, required Ostad to increase the 10-cycle-per-second frequencies. He sat over a hundred feet away, in a separate building. In 75 percent of the patients, brain waves at this frequency increased at the exact moment that Ostad began his healing transmission. In the other 25 percent, the total power in the alpha wave range diminished, indicating some energetic effect.

Another experiment with Ostad measured the stroke volume and cardiac output of the heart, using a very elegant EKG—and related computerized equipment—developed by Dr. Robert Eliot, a well-known cardiologist. In a test of five individuals, again with Ostad positioned more than a hundred feet away in a different room, he was asked to increase cardiac output and stroke volume. There was indeed a marked change in this particular physiological measurement at that time.

In another test, Ostad applied his hands to fifteen sealed plastic bottles of spring water purchased at a regular department store.

Fifteen control bottles were sent away for testing to three different sites for infrared absorption and ultraviolet absorption measures before he applied his healing touch to the next fifteen bottles of water. The "treated" water was then sent for infrared absorption measurements, five bottles each to three separate sites. The results indicated that Ostad's healing energy had significantly affected the molecular structure of water, specifically the hydrogen bonds measured by infrared absorption.

Beginning with my meetings with Olga Worrall, I set out to find medical records proving the efficacy of soul medicine. Ostad Parvarandeh was a treasure trove, leading me to over a hundred medically verifiable accounts of miraculous healing of illnesses ranging from brain tumors and cancer to diabetes. The scientific tests summarized in this book provide further evidence of his abilities. As time goes on, reports are being accumulated of tens of thousands of patients who have been healed by soul medicine, often after being failed by conventional medicine. Flocks of white crows are becoming common!

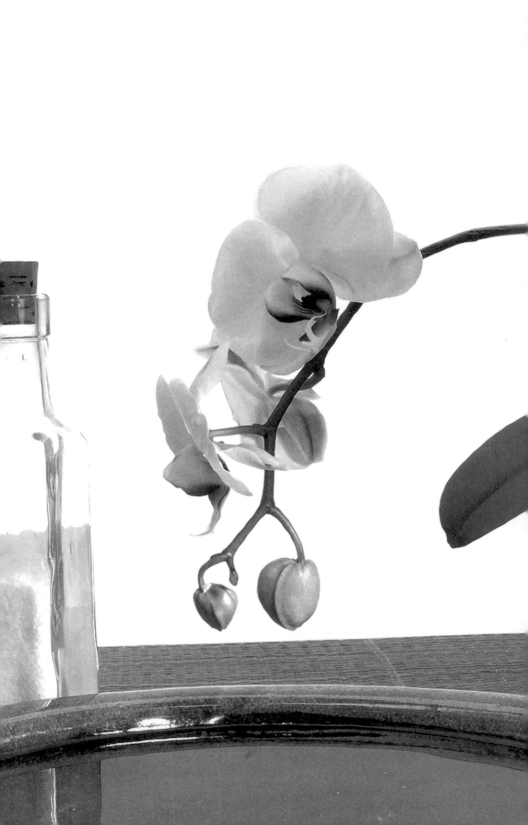

15

Unzipping Chronic and Autoimmune Conditions

Hans Selye began to understand stress when he noted that a number of symptoms were common to most illnesses:

Aches and pains

Looking or feeling unwell

Digestive upsets

Rashes

Fever

Careful observation led him eventually to synthesize these symptoms into a syndrome called stress.[1] Stress is now universally acknowledged to be a factor in virtually all disease, and the cause of many. It's a foundational concept of modern medicine and psychology. Yet before Selye, no-one had forged this durable concept of stress out of this easily observed catalog of symptoms.

Medicine is today confronted by a similar collection of symptoms in need of a common understanding. They include:

Depression

Lethargy

Anxiety

Irritability

Psychological or Emotional Exhaustion

Impaired concentration

Insomnia

Headaches

Aches and pains

These symptoms are common to many of the diseases that have been showing up with increasing frequency in the modern age, such as chronic fatigue syndrome, multiple sclerosis, fibromyalgia, lupus, and thyroid imbalances. These conditions, and others, all have in common an imbalance in the body's electromagnetic field. This may be referred to as Electromagnetic Dysthymia (EMD). EMD is as much a spiritual or existential illness as a physical one. Dr. Herb Benson, who raised the curtain on the mind-body medicine era in the 1970s with his book *The Relaxation Response,* recently observed that: "60 percent to 90 percent of today's medical problems are in the mind-body stress-related realm where the drugs and surgery don't work."[2] Eminent Duke University scientist Ralph Snyderman says, "Most of our nation's investment in health is wasted on an irrational, uncoordinated, and inefficient system that spends more than two-thirds of each dollar treating largely irreversible chronic diseases."[3] Conventional medicine has little to offer EMD suffers; as a group they are particularly motivated to look at the benefits of soul medicine.

Every illness will eventually overload and weaken the adrenal glands, which ordinarily balance the body's stress level. Thus, adrenal burnout, a prominent cause of EMD, is also involved in every major disease. As long as the body can restore homeostasis or natural balance, major disease does not occur and DHEA levels remain reasonably adequate. As adrenal capability fails, DHEA progressively declines, weakening the immune system and reducing one's total life energy.

How does EMD relate to the great diseases of modern society, heart disease, cancer, stroke, and diabetes? Stress is the cumulative pressure that we encounter in going about our daily lives. It is caused by:

- Physical Injuries: fractures, cuts, excess cold or hot
- Chemicals: alcohol, nicotine, caffeine, food additives
- Electromagnetic Fields: radio, TV, computers, cell phones, microwaves
- Mental Habits: worry, frustration
- Emotional Habits: fear, guilt, anger, anxiety, depression
- Spiritual Crises: moral dilemmas, existential anxiety, crises of faith

Illness is the body's reaction to total life stress. EMD is the stress-induced burnout or overload of the body's electromagnetic framework. Illnesses manifest in the organs or systems most strongly associated with that particular stress.

For instance, in the case of coronary artery disease, the dominant influencing factor can be unresolved anger that blocks forgiveness, compassion, love and ultimately the very life force (in this case blood) to the heart itself. A stroke is often associated with the failure to use reason or wisdom. In diabetes, the body's conflict is sometimes related to resentment over having too much or too little responsibility. Cancer is virtually always the end result of intense depression, secondarily focused on the organ or body part involved. For instance, breast cancer can represent depression over a perception of inadequate nurturing. Prostate or uterine cancer likely involves problems of security or sexuality.

235

And so it goes. The electromagnetic deprivation of energy affects the organ or body region with the greatest unresolved emotional distress. Yet it's less important to link every illness with a particular spiritual or emotional malaise, than it is to notice and release emotional and spiritual contractions as soon as possible after they appear. Fear, anxiety, resentment, anger, guilt and depression block life energy.

Diagnosing EMD

The Cornell Medical Index (CMI) was touted a generation ago as adequate for making a clinical diagnosis with 80 percent accuracy, without any need for a person to undergo physical examination or lab tests. The CMI includes family history and past history.

The manifestation of thirty or more symptoms in one person in one year indicates the beginning of the body's failure to cope adequately with stress. Of course, thirty-plus symptoms might be present in a serious illness such as cancer or psychosis, so careful diagnostic testing is required to rule out other treatable illnesses. The list of EMD symptoms includes the following:

- Chronic fatigue
- Immune system problems
- Depression
- Lowered DHEA
- Intracellular magnesium deficiency
- Deficiency of one or more essential amino acids
- EEG brain map abnormalities

These are symptoms of many chronic illnesses. Ultimately EMD is diagnosed when every usual physical illness is ruled out.

Chronic Fatigue Syndrome

Chronic Fatigue Syndrome is simply one extreme of EMD. The

illness typifies EMD, as it relates to stress overload of the adrenal glands. One of the more controversial illnesses of the last decade, the syndrome appears to have existed in the 1800s and was referred to as "neurasthenia." Florence Nightingale probably suffered from it. Other diagnoses have also been used to describe this confusing array of symptoms, including Wilson's disease, chronic Epstein-Barr, candidiasis, environmental sensitivity and myeloencephalopathy.

The prominent symptoms of Chronic Fatigue Syndrome are lack of energy, poor quality sleep, a need for more sleep or rest than normal, anxiety, irritability and weakness. No specific diagnostic test exists for these symptoms. Many treatments produce only transient improvement, if any.

Most of the individuals suffering from Chronic Fatigue Syndrome have probably experienced a major life crisis such as divorce, the death of a loved one, a job or career dislocation, or some other emotionally and spiritually traumatic event that initiated a situational depressive reaction. However, some individuals with this condition have never felt happy. Chronic Fatigue Syndrome may be the physical expression of a disease of the spirit. "Many people in our technological society are disconnected from the matrix of the universe," writes shaman and psychologist Alberto Villoldo. "I often find that people who come to see me with the symptoms of chronic fatigue have become totally disassociated from the natural world. They do not go for walks in the woods, plant tomatoes in their gardens, or even stop to smell the flowers. This is not to say that walking in the forest will cure chronic fatigue syndrome, which is a complex medical condition. Yet people who suffer from this condition require vital reconnection to the natural grid as part of their healing."[4]

Social Contributions to EMD

At some level we all suffer the consequences of negative emotions and behavior. All illness and ultimately death result from cumulative total stress: physical, chemical, emotional, mental, electromagnetic and spiritual. Spiritual distress results, in part, from disregarding

The Golden Rule. Perhaps the most important human lesson is to learn to live that rule consciously, subconsciously, unconsciously and superconsciously, individually and collectively, at all levels of our being. Environmentalists emphasize the negative health effects of pollution. Yet moral, spiritual and psychological pollution may have equally devastating effects. We are affected by the dysfunctions of the society we live in; this generates a constant level of moral tension and background stress. The collective unconscious—the overall energetic field of our society—contains negative influences that all of our immune systems must grapple with. Ervin Lazlo tells us that: "Our body is part of the biosphere and it resonates with the web of life on this planet. And our mind is part of our body, in touch with other minds as well as the biosphere."[5] Researcher William Collinge, in his book *Subtle Energy*, reminds us that "our physical bodies can be influenced by distant attention from others. Researchers have concluded that we are capable of participating with others in a field of events that is transpersonal (beyond the limitations of space or distance), transtemporal (beyond the limitations of time), and transpersonal (beyond what we ordinarily think of as the boundaries between people)."[6] Even when we aim to be healthy, we live in a sea of influences of every time, from the most sublime, to the most destructive ideas and practices of society.

Mahatma Gandhi popularized an awareness of seven types of social sins:

- Politics without principles

- Wealth without work

- Pleasure without conscience

- Knowledge without character

- Science without humanity

- Commerce without morality

- Worship without sacrifice

To Gandhi's list could be added an eighth: intolerance of

normal, healthy, nonharmful behavior! In Springfield, Missouri, "tolerance" was removed from the list of community values, because some religious fundamentalists found the word offensive. They are unwilling to tolerate homosexuality and many other variations of individuality.

At the individual level, evidence of the adverse effects of negative thinking and feeling are convincing to anyone willing to examine the facts. Fear, anxiety, guilt, anger and depression are the major negative emotions. Each of them evokes a stress reaction, more difficult to evaluate than the effects of nicotine, caffeine or alcohol—yet ultimately more insidiously pervasive. These gross emotional reactions are easier to study than the effects of prejudices such as racial or gender discrimination. What are the individual and collective effects of bigotry? What are the physiological effects in a person who is subjected to bigotry? When people such as Mahatma Gandhi or Martin Luther King are struggling for improvement of human behavior, for righting wrongs, is their physiology compensated positively? What are the effects of constant exposure to the suffering of others? Is there a negative drain from being exposed to the anger or depression of others? Did a saint such as Mother Theresa receive physiological benefits as well as spiritual ones from her work with suffering?

We have to live in the society in which we find ourselves. Yet we can still choose our attitudes and actions. The ultimate regulator of brain and mind and, thus, the electromagnetic framework of life is the human spirit. Our knowledge of the effects of anger and depression tells us that you cannot afford the luxury of fear, anxiety, anger, guilt or depression, no matter what the "cause!" And society can't afford prejudice, dislike, hatred, resentment, greed or ignorance (the failure to accept truth or facts). At some level there is a negative physiological effect on the people living in that society. Societies and communities that emphasize caring, connection, cooperation, equality, equanimity, spirituality, joy, tolerance, and love are contributing to the health of their members.

Hormonal and Nutritional Deficiencies and EMD

Much of the medical literature uses the standard that DHEA deficiency is a diagnosis (for men) of less than 180 mg/dL and (for women) less than 130 mg/dL. These standards may be much too low. The mean for each gender is much higher: 715 mg/dL in men and 510 mg/dL in women. DHEA levels below each gender's mean imply progressively diminished adrenal reserve. Most patients with EMD have levels less than 50 percent of the mean, and none have levels at the mean or above. Therefore, DHEA deficiency is common and present in virtually every major illness, as well as in EMD, suggesting relative adrenal exhaustion or adrenal maladaptation.

Magnesium regulates membrane potential, the resting electrical charge on cells. A deficiency of magnesium contributes considerably to the increased sensitivity of patients with EMD. Eighty percent of women and 70 percent of men do not consume the recommended daily intake of magnesium, which should be obtained from eating appropriate amounts of fruits and veggies. Unfortunately our soil is deficient in magnesium so that our food supply is deficient! Rampant magnesium deficiency is associated with most chronic illnesses. Though low intracellular magnesium is not diagnostic of any disease, EMD is inevitably associated with such deficiency.

Malnutrition is also common in many chronic illnesses, particularly in chronically depressed patients. The body's essential amino acids produce most of our neurochemicals. Thus, norepinephrine, serotonin, melatonin and beta-endorphin—all crucial neurochemicals essential for feeling energetic—cannot be properly balanced when there is a deficiency in the amino acid building blocks.

Taurine is now considered an essential amino acid by many scientists. It is deficient in 86 percent of patients with depression. The deficiency of both magnesium and taurine evokes hypersensitivity of cells in patients with EMD. Thus, they have a lower tolerance for many stressors.

The Beginning of a Cure

The EMD malady is much more common than any other disease and indeed is concomitant in many diseases. In its simplest form, EMD results in significant depression. As an individual's ability to cope with increasing stress—including noise, poor nutrition, psychosocial pressures and pollution—is lost, homeostasis becomes erratic and DHEA begins to decrease.

Electromagnetic pollution increasingly contributes to stress. Fluorescent lights, electrical appliances, computers, automobiles, airplanes, radio, television, and microwave emissions bombard the human energy system daily. This may provide major electromagnetic stress.

Sir William Osler believed that there was one common cause of illness. Stress illnesses indicate an electromagnetic overload, leading to a psychoneuroimmunological breakdown. EMD is a factor in virtually all illness. EMD affects the limbic system and hypothalamus, leading to a loss of electrical homeostasis of the brain-mind. EMD illness manifests as depression, with or without a multiple system disease.

The major stress-reduction techniques listed below provide the foundation for therapy. Eighty-five percent of patients respond initially to two weeks of intensive multimodal treatment, and 70 percent improve long-term.

- Photostimulation

- Education

- Music

- Biofeedback

- Guided imagery

- Autogenic training

Recovery may be assisted by magnesium replacement and amino acid supplementation, DHEA restoration, and use of the Liss

CES, Shealy series, transcranially, or the SheLi TENS on the Ring of Fire circuit.

Fear, anger, guilt, anxiety, depression, pessimism, prejudice, hatred, resentment and greed sap or zap our health. What are the antidotes? Joy, laughter, happiness, serenity, peacefulness, optimism, forgiveness, patience, tolerance, compassion and love. These attributes of the spirit enhance health and well-being. They build beta endorphins, the feel-good, natural narcotics, DHEA and immune competency. Cultivating these positive attitudes, emotions and behaviors is a form of soul medicine that anyone can practice. Poets, artists, musicians, novelists and theologians are the doctors reminding us to celebrate the spiritual virtues.

A number of letters from patients with chronic fatigue or depression attest that they consider themselves healed after being treated by sacred healers. Because EMD is a disease primarily of low vital energy, it is a prime example of a spiritual disease. Sufferers can benefit proportionally from soul medicine. Just as allopathic medicine offered many benefits for the medical conditions of the nineteenth and twentieth centuries, soul medicine is well-suited to treating the emerging widespread conditions of the twenty-first century.

SECTION VI

Soul Medicine of the Future

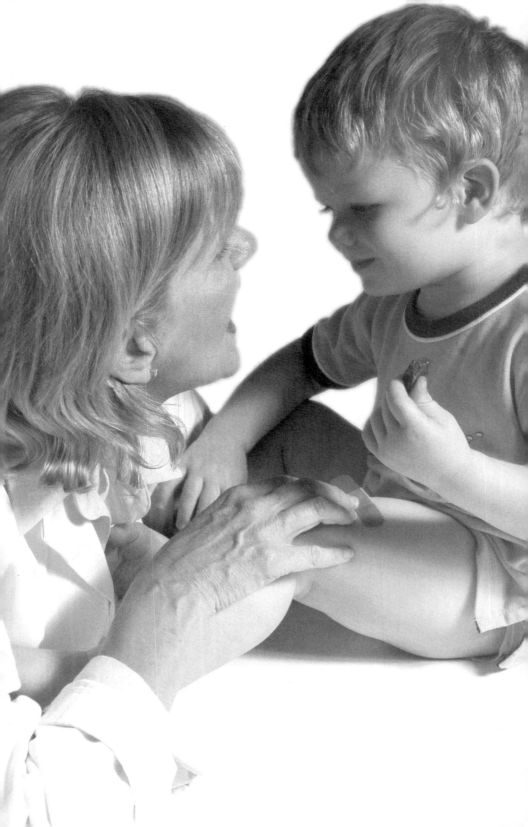

16

How To Find Your Ideal Practitioner

I f you have a condition that needs healing, and you've chosen soul medicine, you have a wealth of potential modalities and practitioners from whom to choose. You have access, through Ayurveda, Chinese Medicine and Shamanism, to therapies that have over twenty times the years of experience that modern Western medicine possesses. You have recourse to treatments like EFT and subconscious programming, which can produce very rapid change. You have options like electrostimulation and Healing Touch, which can improve conditions that baffle allopathic medicine.

Once you've researched soul medicine modalities, you are ready to choose a practitioner, or team of practitioners, to assist you on your healing journey. Making the right choices here can make an enormous difference. There may be only one local practitioner of the method you want to explore, or there may be dozens. It will require some work on your part to narrow your search. What is the best way to approach it?

First, faith in your practitioner is essential. It's even more

245

important, given the nature of soul healing, than the modality you choose. Since we know that most disease results from blockages between soul and body, the method you use to reduce or remove the blockages is less important than the act of removing them. An acupuncturist can help create flow, as can an electromagnetic device. Since the quality of your own intention and belief is the most important single element in your healing, you must have a practitioner who you believe is able to help you effectively.

Second, having an active partnership with your practitioners is a must. You have responsibility for your own well-being, and you are seeking a partner who will assist you in your journey. Choose a practitioner in whom you trust, and with whom you feel comfortable. Communication should feel clear and easy. You should feel a mutual respect. It should be easy to be completely honest with this person. After all, you are forging a relationship between partners, a relationship on which your life may depend. A high-quality relationship creates and alliance to facilitate healing.

It's important to meet your practitioners in person before making final choices. You should feel comfortable in their professional setting. Compare your expectations with theirs. Check in with your body: how do you feel when you are around this person. Are there areas of tightness or strain? What are they trying to tell you?

Check out the background and qualifications of the practitioners you are considering. You will usually find one or more of the following qualifications:

Licensed Professionals

This group includes medical doctors (MDs), osteopaths (DOs), acupuncturists (L.Ac.s), and Nurse Practitioners. The licensing procedure for these professionals is rigorous. After several years of schooling, they are required to pass a stringent exam, and complete a residency program under the supervision of highly experienced clinicians. However, the percentage of these professionals with an integrated, holistically oriented approach is small.

Certified Practitioners

Numerous bodyworkers and energy healers fall into this category. Examples of certification are Certified Massage Therapists (CMTs) and Certified Hypnotherapists (CHTs). Certification standards differ widely from state to state and profession to profession. A certification can mean as little as having completed an eight-hour class, or as much as having 3,000 hours of supervised practice. You can usually find out what's involved in obtaining certification in your state by doing a web search. This will acquaint you with the qualifications of the person from whom you are seeking treatment.

Healers

Healers may have studied a great deal, and worked under the supervision of teacher for many years. Or they may be self-described and self-ordained. They may have unique gifts that fit into no professional category. Most of the healers described in earlier chapters fit this description. They are bona fide spiritual healers whose gifts usually became apparent in childhood. Yet there are also charlatans and con artists in the business of taking advantage of sick people, so it's worth checking out an uncertified practitioner especially closely.

There are also practitioners who are knowledgeable in several fields. It is not uncommon today to find medical doctors who are also certified Ayurvedic physicians, licensed acupuncturists, and licensed Nutritional Doctors (NDs)—all in one. Healers tend to have a lifelong interest in healing, and a curiosity about new approaches. Licensed professionals are also required to obtain continuing education credits, or CEs, each year. Many use this requirement to study an additional modality.

Master Zhi Gang Sha was already a highly respected physician and acupuncturist when he apprenticed himself to Master Guo. He writes: "I earned a medical degree in Western medicine at Xian Jiao Tong Medical University. However, my work as an institutional physician soon revealed that Western medicine was unable to help many patients. I realized that integrating it with traditional Chinese medicine would combine the best of both systems, so I obtained certification as a doctor of traditional Chinese medicine. [Then] I became a disciple of Dr. Zhi Chen Guo. Under Master Guo's rigorous training...my spiritual channels were opened, and I became a medical intuitive."[1]

A healer may have studied a particular modality but not have the experience to treat you in depth; in such cases ethical practitioners recognize the limits of their expertise and will certainly refer you to a highly competent specialist. Throughout this book, and in the appendices, you will find the names of healers we recommend you investigate.

Referrals and Office Visits

Once you've checked out the qualifications of a potential healing partner, ask for referrals. Most healing professionals will supply you with the names of past patients who can vouch for their work. And your coworkers, family members, friends and social contacts are sources of possible information. Your primary care physician may have suggestions for soul medicine practitioners, and may surprise you with his or her knowledge of the field. Patients groups, support groups, and professional societies can supply you with information. Most colleges have lists of their practicing alumni online. Groups like the American Holistic Medical Association (www.AHMA.com) and the American Board of Scientific Medical Intuition (www.ABSMI.org) make their practitioner lists available online, and you will find many others in almost every specialty with the aid of a web search engine.

Practitioner web sites are also a good source of information. Their web sites will often tell you their credentials, professional affiliations, training, how many years they've been practicing, treatment philosophy, endorsements and testimonials, details of their particular techniques, and what you can expect during the course of a professional relationship.

Use a search engine and type in the practitioner's name. This will give you a list of their publications, recent news stories about them, web sites on which they're listed, and a host of details. Patient complaints will often show up here; there are sites that allow people to let off steam about bad experiences.

Payment information is usually not on a practitioner's web site, and you will usually have to call their office to find that out. A few operate within HMO, PPO or other medical insurance plans; most do not. Many offer a sliding scale based on financial ability. Some offer a free or low-cost introductory visit or examination.

Use your intuition. Remember that your 11+ million bit-per-second subconscious scanning computer is already doing the evaluation! Draw on its wisdom. An initial consultation, armed with the right questions, will give you a sense of whether this is the right healing partner for you.

In the course of that initial consultation, be completely frank with your prospective partner. Describe all aspects of your life that might be relevant to your health concern. Make your expectations explicit. Ask the practitioner for a frank assessment of your future prospects with them. If anything the person says doesn't sound right, let them know, and take note of how they handle the interaction. Are they able to accept feedback? Notice the person's experience and intelligence level as well as the feel-good factors; there are highly empathetic practitioners who are not very effective, and geniuses are often short of manner, and intolerant of lesser talents.

Find out whether they will keep written records, and whether they will share them with other healing partners. Find out how long they estimate your treatment might take. Make notes, after the interview, of your observations, both positive and negative. If you don't already keep a journal, a healing journey is a great opportunity to start one. Practitioner interviews will focus you on tuning into your body and intuitive wisdom, as well as your intellectual observations.

Get an accurate diagnosis. This might take visits to several different practitioners. But the time and expense required is virtually always worthwhile. An accurate diagnosis is an essential first step in treatment. For some conditions, especially those related to EMD, a conventional allopathic diagnosis might be difficult to obtain. But a visit to a good diagnostician can certainly rule out obvious organic causes of disease.

Supplementing a *diagnosis* by a licensed professional is the possibility of an *assessment*. An assessment is done by a healer; rather than aiming to identify a disease, it targets an area of energy blockage. The site of the blockage may be far from the site of symptoms, and precede any symptoms at all. Daniel Benor, M.D., a distinguished researcher who was the first to systematically catalog scientific studies that supported the role of spirituality in healing, drew this distinction in a paper entitled *Intuitive Assessments: An Overview*. He writes: "Reports abound of healers identifying problems present in healees. Many healers are able to intuit where to place their hands in order to give healing. Healees often comment on the fact that healers "find the right spot" without being told.... Some healers feel or see the biological energy fields around people and are guided by their sense of touch or by the colors of the energy field to places that need healing.... I have spoken with hundreds of healers and healees over two decades of healing explorations. I cannot count the numbers of stories I have heard of chronic pains, fevers, and diseases that eluded medical diagnosis and were clarified through intuitive assessments."[2]

Once you start treatment, remember the partnership model. You and the practitioner or practitioners are a team, committed to your healing. Be proactive. Ask questions. Challenge suggestions that you don't understand, or that feel wrong to you. Share disappointments as well as triumphs. Talk about your expectations openly. Get your practitioner's e mail address so that you can communicate in this way too, and find out how often he or she checks and responds to e mails. But don't impose, expecting your practitioner to substitute long free e mail conversations for office visits. They do not have the time.

Let all the members of your healing team know what's happening.

You might set up an online group to share information; several portals like Yahoo, Google and MSN have "group" services that take just a few minutes to set up. Having a group like "GeorgeGoringHealing@ yahoogroups.com"—and entering the e mail addresses of all those on your healing team, allows a comment sent by any practitioner to go to all. Again, take care about e mail contact. It's like a hot line: used sparingly, it can be vital. If you overuse it, your healing professionals will tend to ignore your communications in this format.

Keep your primary care physician informed about other treatments. Patients often make the mistake of thinking that herbs must be safe because they're natural. But some herbs have adverse reactions when used with certain drugs. And drugs can inhibit the effectiveness of some herbal formulations. Your ND, who may be prescribing herbs, needs to know what your MD, who may be prescribing drugs, is doing, and vice versa. An informed treatment team is an effective treatment team.

Sometimes even the smartest patient simply cannot understand some aspect of treatment. You might feel foolish asking, or asking again—and again.

Do it anyway. Healing professionals have their own mindsets and jargon. They may think they're being perfectly clear, and the course of treatment might indeed be routine and simple to them. But it's new to you, and it might take you a while to understand aspects of it. So nodding your head when you can't follow the conversation is a bad idea. Ask till you're sure you understand what's going on—it's an essential part of taking responsibility for your own well-being. You are your best physician. One of the most wonderful integrative, holistic physicians, Dr. Gladys McGarey, often speaks of the physician within. If you realize that your problems are primarily the result of unresolved emotional stress, you will find a complete self-therapy program is *Ninety Days to Stress-Free Living*, a guide to nurturing yourself.[3]

Use your journal to track the results of your treatment. Evaluate how you're doing. Have the patience to give each treatment time to have its effect. Some produce very quick results. Some may result in you feeling worse before you feel better. Getting in touch with your body—and really being present to the dysfunction that you've been pushing to the back of your mind for the last five years—may result in you feeling worse. Holistic health aims to treat the whole person, rather than aiming a magic bullet at a particular pain. Your practitioner may treat a site a long way from the pain. Soul medicine looks for the root problem, rather than trying to make the symptom go away. Your practitioner can usually give you an average time it has historically taken other patients with your condition to get well—your healing time may be more or less. It may take patience, and learning patience is an essential part of a healing journey. The Old Testament tells the story of Naaman, head of the mighty Syrian army. He developed leprosy, and his body was covered with sores. His healing instruction was to, "Go and wash in Jordan [river] seven times, and thy flesh shall come again to thee, and thou shalt be clean." Naaman, an impatient overachiever, "was wroth, and...went away in a rage." He had many better ideas of how his healing might be accomplished. Yet when he finally learned patience, and went along with the program, "his flesh came again like unto the flesh of a little child,"[4] and he was healed. So give the process time, and keep an open mind.

A healing partnership involves both information and intuition. Illness is an opportunity to become exquisitely conscious, to straddle both worlds, to be fully in your body, as well as fully present with your spirit. It is a chance to find out about advanced treatments, as well as using common sense. Healing is a milestone on your spiritual journey. Embrace it as a powerful spiritual teacher!

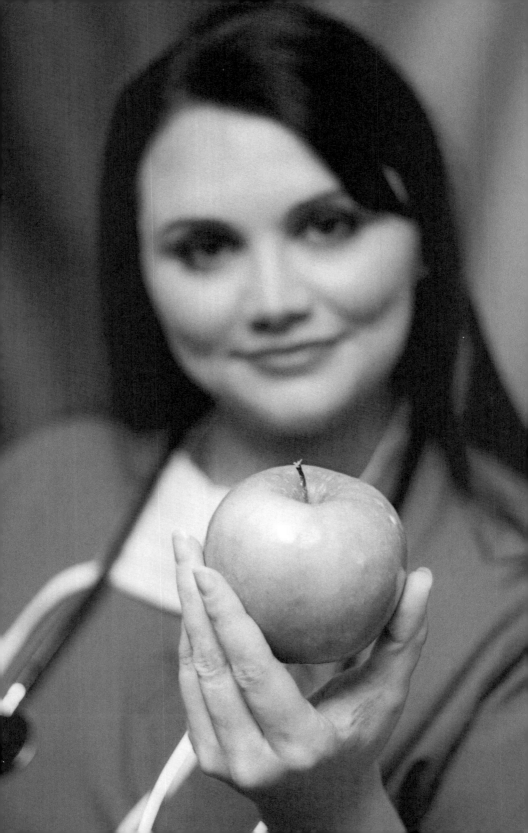

17

Mainstreaming Soul Medicine

S ociety is heavily invested in the current medical system. Despite its failure to keep people well, to develop safe and non-invasive techniques, and to study promising therapies outside of the consensus biomedical model, our social system continues to fund and support allopathic medicine to the hilt.

Allopathic medicine and research now accounts for some 15 percent of the Gross National Product of the United States. Duke University's Ralph Snyderman recently declared that we spend, "well over a trillion dollars a year on acute episodes of late-stage chronic diseases, which in many instances are not reversible."[1] That's half of America's health care budget. "This year, General Motors will spend more on health care for employees and pensioners than on steel," said Arkansas governor Mike Huckabee in 2006.[2]

On cancer research and treatment, since President Nixon declared a War on Cancer, some two trillion dollars has been spent. For those of us suffering from "zero shock," that's *two thousand billion* dollars, or *two hundred thousand* million dollars. Despite this astonishing allocation of national resources, the percentage of Americans dying from cancer (adjusted for age) is about the same as it was in 1950. A recent report notes that long-term survival rates from common cancers such as breast, prostate, colorectal and lung cancer has barely budged since the 1970s.[3] An editorial from Richard Smith in the *British Medical Journal* reminds us that "only 15 percent of medical interventions are supported by solid scientific evidence," and that "This is because only 1 percent of the articles in medical journals are scientifically sound, and partly because many treatments have never been assessed at all."[4]

A study of the Gerson method of alternative cancer treatment, an approach that relies on frequent preparation of very fresh vegetables, and the elimination of virtually all toxins, evaluated the five year survival rates of 153 melanoma patients. It found that 100 percent of the patients with Stage One and Stage Two cancers receiving the Gerson therapy survived, but only 70 percent of the conventionally treated patients. For patients with cancer that had spread to other sites close to the original cancer (Stage Three) seventy percent of the Gerson patients survived, versus 41 percent of those treated with allopathic medical techniques. Of those patients whose cancer had spread to distant parts of their body (Stage Four), 39 percent of the Gerson patients were still alive, compared to just 6 percent of those treated with conventional therapy.[5] This kind of result is astounding; there were *six* patients alive on the Gerson treatment for every *one* patient receiving conventional chemotherapy and radiation.

Dartmouth Medical School did a study that examined death rates among patients recovering from heart surgery. They found that the survival rate of people who possessed a strong foundation in their religious faith, and a vibrant social network, had *fourteen* times the survival rate of those who did not. "A Yale University study of 28,212 elderly people found that those who rarely or never attended church had *twice* the stroke rate of weekly churchgoers." Another study of older adults in Marin County, California, showed that those who attended religious services weekly—even occasionally—were 36 percent less likely to die after procedures than those that did not.[6]

A promising series of studies has been done on the fruit and wood of the paw paw tree by researchers at Purdue University. This plant contains acetogenins, which affect the production of ATP in the mitochondrial powerhouses of cancer cells, and reduces the growth of the capillaries that sustain cancer. It is also the only compound proven effective against MDR or Multiple Drug Resistant cells in breast cancer.[7] Purdue University has done several similar studies, but these and the Gerson study described above are among the very, very few properly-conducted studies comparing alternative natural therapies with conventional treatments for cancer.

We have heard hundreds of anecdotal accounts from patients who have healed themselves using visualization, prayer, faith healing, electromagnetic stimulation, homeopathy, biofeedback, lifestyle changes, superior nutrition, emotional healing, herbs, meridian-based therapies, and other forms of soul medicine.

One of those patients whose story stands out is Nancy. She was diagnosed in 1972 with Stage Four cervical cancer. Her cancer had metastasized to several other sites in her body. She was given only a few months to live by her doctor.

Nancy's diagnosis occurred when there were no cancer support groups, when alternative treatments were being vigorously suppressed, when alternative cancer clinics were being outlawed, when alternative therapists were being jailed, when research was scarce and hard to perform, and when there were no books or articles on surviving the grim statistics for metastatic cancer.

She'd heard of a technique called creative visualization. She could not bear the thought of going through the prescribed course of chemotherapy and radiation. An exceptionally strong willed human being, she reasoned: "My body created this thing, so my body has the power to uncreate it, too." She decided to try creative visualization for herself.

She left work, and began to do nothing except take care of herself. She rested, did what exercise her exhausted state would allow, and ate and drank more carefully. She visualized the cancer cells being eaten up by little white stars in her body. She imagined the stars falling through her body many times a day. Each time one of the points of a star touched a cancer cell, it punctured the cell. The cell died, and the remains dribbled out of her body.

She would lie in a bath for hours, and imagined the cancer cells being washed away by the stars. She filled her mind with little except self-nurturing, and little white stars.

She began to feel better and better. Her walks became longer. Her appetite increased. Her focus slowly began to shift from immediate survival, and she began to picture a future for herself. She started to dream of what goals she might pursue in the next few years.

After three months, she returned to her doctor, feeling vibrantly healthy. She was tested, but had no anxiety about the outcome. When the test results came back, her doctor was astonished; she was completely cancer-free, as she knew she would be. She was still sharing her story with other people more than ten years afterwards. Nancy was still in excellent health, and the cancer had not returned.

Such images are highly personal, and work best when the patient comes up with images that speak potently to both conscious and subconscious mind. Another man visualized "'white-immune-cell bunny rabbits feasting on fields of orange cancer carrots.' A particularly fascinating part of these elaborate imageries is that some of those who created them seemed to know prior to medical discovery that their cancer was gone. One morning the man with the immune-cell bunny rabbits 'couldn't find enough carrots for all my rabbits.' Shortly thereafter, his physician reported the cancer gone."[8]

Society's ignorance of soul medicine is very costly. Billions of dollars lost in the form of sick days and underperforming employees. In the US the figures for economic losses are huge: Persistent pain costs the US economy an estimated $100 billion per year in medical bills, lost tax revenue, welfare and disability payments, and lost productivity by workers who are on the job but in pain.[9] According to the *Journal of the American Medical Association,* the latter factor alone, "presenteeism," costs the US economy some 61 billion dollars per year.[10] Occasioning some 40 million doctor visits each year, pain is the most common reason behind medical appointments.[11] Chronic pain patients have, on average, complained of pain for seven years, undergone three major surgeries, and incurred medical bills of between $50,000 and $100,000.[12] The British health ministry estimates that 11 million work days are lost in Great Britain each year because of back pain alone.[13] This is a condition from which, at the Shealy Institute, we have found that 50 percent of patients, find relief using an inexpensive TENS device and another 35 percent benefit from the broader soul medicine approach.

During brain surgery videotaped for Bill Moyers' PBS documentary *Healing and the Mind,* a patient scheduled for brain surgery did not receive general anesthesia as would have been mandatory under the allopathic model. Instead, the patient received only an acupuncture treatment for pain. The patient remained awake and pain-free during the brain surgery procedure, and was even able to converse with the attending medical staff.[14] Coauthor Norman Shealy performed such surgery with TENS devices in the late 1960s. Such results point to efficacy using soul medicine that is completely beyond the reach of allopathic medicine.

In a landmark study of wound healing, deep incisions were made on the shoulders of twenty-three male college students. The experimental group received Therapeutic Touch, in which the hands of the healer are held over the wound and energy directed toward its healing. The control group did not receive energy healing. At an early point in the study, the wounds of the students in the Therapeutic Touch group were 94 percent healed. In the control group, the wounds were 67 percent healed.[15] Experiments like this show dramatic results from energy medicine techniques—results that cannot be explained by any biomedical model. A large scale study of studies performed between the beginning of 1999 and the end of 2004 recently compared the cost-effectiveness of conventional medical treatments with CAM alterative treatments. Because of the limited number of studies done on alternatives, the number of conditions they could compare for were limited. However, they found that CAM treatments were more cost-effective than conventional medicine every time; for Parkinson's disease, for migraines, for neck pain, for stress management, for IBS (irritable bowel syndrome), and for other conditions.[16]

You would assume that, given the success of soul medicine and alternative therapies for cancer, pain, and wound healing, society would be busily redirecting a huge proportion of that two trillion dollars into soul medicine based approaches. You would assume that scientists would be energetically studying people like Nancy, in a focused effort to understand where this magic comes from.

And you would be wrong. The Gerson study mentioned above is one of only a handful comparing conventional cancer treatment with alternative therapies. Just a few million dollars a year are spent on soul medicine research, less than one percent of what is spent on conventional treatment.

If we take as a starting point the National Institutes of Health figure that patients spend $34 billion a year on complementary and alternative medicine (CAM), and that the total health care expenditures of the US are about $1.8 trillion annually, this means that CAM represents less than .02 percent of medical spending. This ratio, with allopathic care receiving 99.8 percent of funding, and CAM receiving just a tiny sliver, represents a severe imbalance.

Our society is like a man trying to improve an engine. He's been spending a thousand dollars a year for half a century on the enterprise. He's believed he is on the verge of a breakthrough many times, but his engine functions at about the same level of efficiency as it did when he began his tinkering fifty years before.

He spends twenty bucks and ninety minutes on a brief experiment called the Gerson engine. He discovers that it works six times better than his existing engine. He raises his eyebrows in surprise. Then he shrugs his shoulders, sets it aside, and goes back to spending a thousand dollars a year on his failed endeavor.

"Modern medicine," observes Larry Dossey, "has become one of the most spiritually malnourished professions in our society.... Because we have so thoroughly disowned the spiritual component of healing, most healers throughout history would view our profession today as inherently perverse. They would be aghast at how we have squeezed the life juices and the heart out of our calling."[17] Thomas McKeown, a British professor of social medicine, brought to our attention that only 8 percent of the longevity gain in the recent centuries can be attributed to the "miracles" of modern science. Instead, pasteurization of milk, chlorination of water, improved sewage control and better nutrition contributed the remaining 92 percent gain.[18] While modern medicine has done little to increase longevity and perhaps even less to enhance the quality of life, soul medicine holds out the promise of both. Yet progress in changing society's focus, in order to shift the ratio of research and treatment dollars in the direction of effective soul medicine treatments is agonizingly slow. Many people are dying, and suffering unnecessarily, in the interim. The pendulum is starting to swing in the other direction, but gradually.

Accreditation Standards for Soul Medicine Practitioners

One factor we believe will accelerate the pace of change is a commonly accepted accreditation program for soul medicine practitioners. Accreditation gives patients the confidence of knowing that a practitioner has received a basic training that encompasses a defined suite of skills, and has passed a basic competency test.

U.S. physicians accomplished this a century and a half ago with the establishment of the American Medical Association in 1847. Two hundred and fifty delegates, hailing from twenty-eight states, were present at the initial meeting at the Academy of Natural Sciences in Philadelphia, Pennsylvania. At this first meeting, the delegates elected Dr. Nathaniel Chapman as president. They adopted a code of medical ethics, as well as a national standard for pre-medical education, and guidelines for the degree of M.D. The prestigious

Journal of the American Medical Association published its first issue in 1883.[19] Psychologists emulated them, with the formation of the American Psychological Association (APA) in 1892, but it was not until the acquisition by the APA board of the journals published by Princeton University psychology professor Howard Warren in the mid 1920s, including *Psychological Review* and the *Journal of Experimental Psychology,* that the APA began to speak with a coherent voice. When the Flexner report destroyed most competition to the allopathic model, the AMAs methods became the dominant modality of treatment.

The chiropractic profession began the process when the educational director of the American Chiropractic Association, John Nugent, began prodding the heads of chiropractic colleges in the 1950s to raise their standards to the levels required for federal accreditation. He first made contact with the United States Office of Education in 1952. Gradually, instructors in the basic sciences were required to have an advanced degree, and a two-year liberal arts college requirement was required as an admission standard. In 1971, under the leadership of Dr. George Haynes, the ACA separately chartered its education committee as the Council on Chiropractic Education (CCE). After a sustained effort, in 1974 the CCE received a letter from the US Commissioner of Education stating that it would be added to the "list of nationally recognized accrediting agencies and associations." At that time there were 4,812 students enrolled in US chiropractic colleges. The largest of these was the oldest, Palmer College, with 1,965 students, and the smallest, Northwestern College, with 130 students. Other than Palmer, no college had more than 600 students.[20] Meanwhile, chiropractic was fighting a running legal battle with the AMA, which was seeking to outlaw chiropractic. The AMA, however, was forced to settle in federal antitrust cases by chiropractors in 1978, 1980, 1986, and 1990.

Soul medicine finds itself in a similar position today. The balance of research dollars and institutional momentum is clearly with the established medical profession. Yet soul medicine treatments are gaining increasing currency among consumers and medical professionals alike. In Philadelphia, the same city that witnessed the founding of the AMA, the University of Pennsylvania has partnered with an alternative medicine school, Tai Sophia Institute, in a program to teach medical students about CAM. According to the Association of American Medical Colleges, more than 95 of the nation's 125 medical schools require some kind of coursework in CAM.[21] With consumers now spending so much money each year out of their own pockets to cover the costs of alternative therapies not covered by their health insurance plans, it's become essential that medical doctors be informed about them.

In addition to the accreditation of individual practitioners through a national board licensing program such as the one that currently exists for holistic MDs, we believe that the accreditation of the educational institutions that train soul medicine practitioners is an essential early step. Holos University Graduate Seminary, in which both coauthors of this book are involved, is in the midst of accreditation proceedings. It is one of several training institutions offering course work in sacred healing; it is striking that their numbers and composition mirror the breakdown of chiropractic colleges thirty years ago.

We are advocating the establishment of an internationally recognized common degree, such as an Energy Medicine Diploma, an EMD. We are suggesting a common set of professional ethics. We are also calling for the establishment of an accrediting agency for institutions offering soul medicine courses. A student would become a diplomate in energy medicine once they have completed the requirements for graduation at an accredited school, which would include a basic curriculum of 60 graduate hours—roughly four full-time semesters—and a substantial practicum. After a board certified written and oral test, and a residency period, they would be licensed for the clinical practice of soul medicine. To be admitted into an EMD program, a student would be required to have completed at least two undergraduate years (60 credits) or be certified as a registered nurse or physician's assistant from an institution accredited by an agency recognized by the US Secretary of Education. These courses could be taken at a variety of institutions, each teaching the subjects they know best, and networked into a single program administered by the accrediting agency for soul medicine.

Here's what a set of required courses might look like:

1. Anatomy and Physiology

A conventional review of the structure and function of the human body. Particular emphasis on signaling systems: biochemical, neural, endocrinal, electromagnetic, and kinesthetic.

2. Soul Medicine Modalities

An overview of all the soul medicine modalities, along with a list of the principles of each, and scientific studies that demonstrate the applications and limitations of each. Demonstrations of each one when possible. Modalities may include: aromatherapy, homeopathy, light and color therapy, kinesiology, electrotherapy, acupuncture, healing touch, prayer, spiritual energetics, and the biochemistry of nutrition.

3. Human Energy Anatomy

An examination of the characteristics of the human bioenergy systems, noting how they interact, and what therapies can be applied to each. The link between physical, emotional, psychological and spiritual interventions. The chakra system. Somatic psychology and therapies. Demonstrations by qualified professional practitioners.

4. Neurology, Psychology, Immunity, and Gene Expression

Energy systems interact with physical structures in various ways, especially through the immune system, emotional states, intentions and beliefs. This course reviews how genes express when influenced by these systems, and gives students a grasp of the fundamentals of psychoneuroimmunology.

5. History of Soul Medicine—Eastern, Western and Indigenous

All societies have developed cultures of healing. These, however, differ from society to society. This course, while examining healing practices in various societies, also will consider what patterns they have in common. This course introduces students to the various systems of integrative health care found in all parts of the world. Western holistic standards, requirements and expectations are reviewed. Indigenous spiritual healing traditions are explained, including Brazilian, Chinese, Hawaiian, Ayurvedic, and Native American.

6. Medical Intuition

Students study the many personal blocks that prevent their natural intuitive ability. They are introduced to ways to change how they receive, react, and adapt to stressful situations, all of which may inhibit intuitive impressions. The course includes personalizing and tuning one's own style of intuition. Practical applications of intuition will be explored through a variety of intuitive exercises. Students then learn how to recognize and facilitate dialogue not only with their own bodies, but those of others. Students learn the foundation skills and application of Body Scanning and its relationship to basic physiology. They then practice their skills against known medical diagnoses in actual case histories.

7. Soul Medicine and Recent Science

A review of statistical methods in research, an evaluation of the quality of research, and a listing of research sources and databases, followed by investigation of some of the most recent publications, scholars and institutions performing research.

8. Energy Psychology

Students learn to understand how the body receives, transmits, and processes emotions, and how anger, sadness, guilt, anxiety, and depression play an important role in our growth. The link between consciousness and emotional processes is emphasized, with the understanding that disease may be a powerful catalyst for change. Meridian-based energy psychology techniques such as EMDR, Shiatsu, EFT and TAT are taught, and the student receives depth instruction of one of the Energy Psychology techniques.

9. Ethical Standards for Soul Medicine Practitioners

Review of the ethical standards governing each modality, and of a unified statement of professional ethics for soul medicine. Awareness of the importance of holistic practice, treating the entire patient. The value of a diagnosis, and cases in which a diagnosis is difficult. An understanding of drug interactions, and the interaction of drugs with herbal formulations and naturopathic treatments. Authoritative sources of professional information. Asking for explicit permissions to work on the patient's energy systems. Ethical marketing, financial and business practices. Maintaining professional boundaries.

10. Practicum

The goal of the advanced practicum is to permit the student to demonstrate professional competency in addressing a particular method soul medicine under the direction of the instructor and guidance of an approved sponsor at the field study site. Students complete a daily journal and prepare a scholarly paper summarizing their findings for the field study. The field study may also consist of a pilot research project in preparation for thesis or dissertation research.

Licensing Board and Residency

Once the student has completed a course of study at an accredited institution that includes these ten classes, or a similar consensus of courses, the student would sit for a board examination, which would consist of a written and an oral examination. The written examination would be in the form of a standardized test that adequately assesses a student's grasp of all the areas of knowledge in the above courses.

Finally a student for the Energy Medicine Diploma would need to pass an oral examination by a group of examiners. At that point, the EMD would be permitted to practice under the supervision of another licensed professional for a period of time—a residency—prior to being licensed and entering into independent clinical practice. Until there are a sufficient number of licensed EMDs under which residents can practice, and even past that point, residents could be supervised by licensed professionals from other professions, such as MDs, DOs, and L.Ac.s (Licensed Acupuncturists). The American Board of Scientific Medical Intuition certifies both Medical Intuitives and Counseling Intuitives who pass such an examination.

This plan fits neatly into existing curricula, and is flexible enough to accommodate both existing universities and students already enrolled in graduate and post-graduate degree programs. These classes could be completed *during the course of* getting a doctorate or a master's degree at a university. Most of the above courses are already part of the core requirements for an advanced degree at Holos and other institutions. So a student would graduate with both a doctorate and an EMD.

This plan is also flexible enough to permit specialization in almost any modality. An EMD could graduate from a school of acupuncture. That would give the practitioner not just a primary treatment method in the form of acupuncture, but a wide grasp of the entire field of soul medicine, and how different modalities can combine for effective complementary treatment. Such a graduate would be both an EMD and an L.Ac. An EMD might alternatively choose a course of study, or an accredited school that focuses on aromatherapy or applied kinesiology, and graduate with a specialization in that field. Such a graduate would be both an EMD and an Applied Kinesiologist.

As holders of EMD degrees provide successful treatment of patients, contribute to clinical studies, serve on the faculties of institutions, lecture at professional conferences, publish research in peer-reviewed professional journals, and write books expanding the scope of professional knowledge, the field of soul medicine will gain in credibility and visibility. Research dollars and publicity should follow, and the promise of soul medicine to alleviate or cure many conditions poorly served by allopathic medicine will be realized.

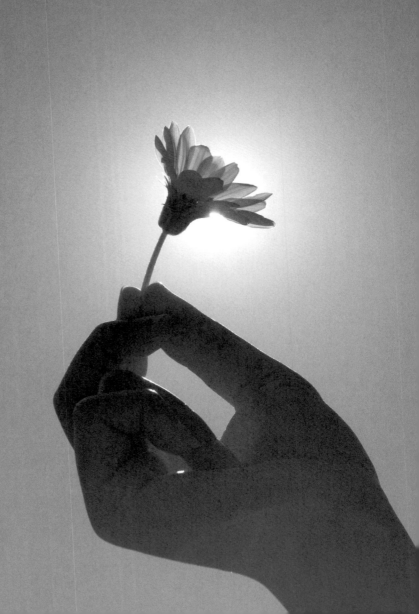

18

Soul: Medicine of the Future

Hugo Munsterberg, a psychologist colleague of William James's, wrote, in 1899: "Our time longs for a new synthesis—it waits for science to satisfy our higher needs for a view of the world that shall give unity to our scattered experience." Science today is giving soul medicine, the principle that unifies so many forms of healing, a validation that would have seemed impossible a few years ago. "For centuries," James Oschman says, "concepts of 'life force' and 'healing energy' have been at the center of one of the most bitter and acrimonious debates in the history of science.... To realize the inestimable promise of electromagnetic medicine, we must overcome the legacy of past dogmas and intolerances, and our fears of invisible forces. How rapidly this takes place depends on each of us... Certainly, for a culture that has become accustomed to having large numbers of tasks handled by invisible currents flowing through chips in computers...it is not too frightening to look at the ways our bodies are regulated and coordinated by invisible energies."[1] Science is now pushing us irresistibly toward overcoming past fears of soul medicine, as study after study points us toward its efficacy.

This has affected the belief systems of some scientists. In an article entitled "Spirituality Soars Among Scientists," that appeared in

271

late 2005 in *Science and Theology News,* writer Lea Plante summarized the findings of a research study by postdoctoral fellow Elaine Ecklund at Rice University. It surveyed over 1,600 scientists from 21 institutions. Ecklund used indicators such as yoga, meditation, scripture reading, and prayer to measure spirituality. Contrary to popular stereotypes of science as an atheistic profession, she found that spirituality "is important to a majority of scientists in the United States' elite research universities." As a result of the mounting scientific evidence for the efficacy of soul healing, direct experience of the divine, and the increasingly spiritual orientation of contemporary society, the number of "spiritual scientists" is increasing. This will have the effect of increasing the spiritual component of future research, and making medicine and society more aware of the empirical basis of soul medicine.[2]

Tom Janisse, M.D., publisher of Kaiser Permanente's *The Permanente Journal,* reports that, "The Permanente Group's physician health department created an educational videotape entitled 'Mindfulness in Medicine,' which focuses on mindfulness practice for busy doctors and health care professionals. Clinicians explain how focusing on breathing and body awareness, responding nonjudgmentally, and feeling less controlled by time improves their work and personal satisfaction."[3] Prayer, meditation, and other consciousness practices are becoming widespread in the healing professions.

The prevalence of prayer amongst physicians today is startling. A study done by the Jewish Theological Seminary in December of 2004 and included 1,087 physicians. Among the doctors were practitioners of many faiths: Catholics, Protestants, Jews (broken out into groups of Orthodox, Conservative, Reform, and culturally identified but not observant Jews), Muslims, Hindus and Buddhists.

The survey found that some two thirds of the doctors surveyed believed that prayer was important, and that three quarters of them believe that miracles occur today. In every group, with the sole exception of less religiously observant Jews, over 50 percent of the physicians believed that miracles occur today. In some groups, like Orthodox Jews and Christians of all stripes, 80 percent or more of the physicians polled believed that miracles happen today.

Two thirds said that they encouraged their patients to pray, either because they believed it was psychologically beneficial to the patient, or because they believed that God might answer those prayers, or both. Half of them said that they encouraged their patients to have other people pray for them. Half of them said that they prayed for their patients as a whole, and almost sixty percent said that they pray for individual patients. An average of fifty-five percent of the physicians reported seeing miraculous recoveries in patients, and a third or more of physicians (of every religious group) said they had seen miraculous recoveries—even when the percentage of doctors in that group who prayed for patients was well below one-third.[4] Prayer has arrived in the consulting room and hospital in force.

One of the striking findings of this poll is that between 50 and 80 percent of physicians, even those of weak religious faith, believe that miracles can happen today. There are many accounts of sudden and dramatic improvement in health, but it is not a well-studied phenomenon, since these tend to be viewed as anomalous phenomena. In their book *Catastrophe Theory,* Alexander Woodcock and Monte Davis note that, "The mathematics underlying three hundred years of science, though powerful and successful, have encouraged a one-sided view of change. These mathematical principles are ideally suited to analyze—because they were created to analyze—smooth, continuous quantitative change: the smoothly curving paths of planets around the sun, the continuously varying pressure of a gas as it is heated and cooled, the quantitative increase of a hormone level in the bloodstream. But there is another kind of change, too, change that is less suited to mathematical analysis: the abrupt bursting of a bubble, the discontinuous transition from ice at its melting point to water at its freeing point, the qualitative quantum shift in our minds when we 'get' a pun or a play on words."[5]

The change offered by soul medicine treatments can seem

miraculous to the old model of healing. Patients can snap out of depression, experience rapid remission of cancer, recover quickly from traumatic injuries, shed childhood wounds in moments, and gain energy overnight. Our old models are good at working with the tiny part of the spectrum of healing they represent. Yet they do not have the sensory range to perceive most of the colors in the spectrum. They break down when confronted with miracles. Like a blind person in an art museum, they hear only the squeak of other patrons' shoes on the polished floor, and their gasps of wonder. They have no basis in which to comprehend the phenomena occurring around them.

Soul medicine is not visible only from the birds-eye view of a treatment professional; the general public has caught on to its efficacy in a big way. The largest and most comprehensive study done to date, reported in 2005 by the National Institutes of Health, surveyed some 31,000 American adults. It found that 36 percent of them had used complementary and alternative medicine (CAM) in the preceding twelve months. But when prayer was included in the definition of CAM, the figure rose to 62 percent.[6] Soul medicine is becoming part of the fabric of medical care and public awareness to a degree not seen for five centuries. James Gordon, a member of the White House Commission on CAM policy, coauthored a report that he hopes "will exercise as profound an effect on twenty-first century medicine" as the Flexner report did on the twentieth. In it, an expert panel advocates, in addition to conventional medicine, for "non-M.D. training programs in 'complementary and alternative' approaches— among them chiropractic, acupuncture, naturopathy, herbalism, and massage therapy. Congressional legislation, supported by an extraordinary bipartisan coalition, reflects the breadth and power of this movement. Rigorous NIH-funded research on therapies that were ignored and disparaged 10 or even 5 years ago is proceeding apace at many of our leading academic medical institutions." The report recommends "legislative initiatives that will make the best of these therapies, and training in them, an integral part of medical and other professional education.

Within a few years, the picture we've painted of the promise of soul medicine will be more than an inspiring vision. It will be an established reality. Today we look at a faded glass sepia photograph of a Civil War surgeon, sawing off shattered limbs with a lumber saw—minus anesthesia—and shudder. We marvel at how medicine ever coped without MRIs, EKGs, penicillin, and quinine.

Yet by the middle of the next decade, we'll look back and shudder at procedures considered normal today. We'll marvel at the barbarity of radical masectomy, the superstition of antidepression treatments, the primitiveness of chemotherapy, the futility of extended psychotherapy, and the ignorance implicit in long-term use of anti-inflammatory drugs. It will amaze us that cures for autoimmune diseases once eluded medicine. It will seem remarkable that patients once abandoned responsibility for their health to harried, overworked and impersonal HMOs.

We will have an array of new tools at our disposal: non-invasive energy healing techniques that can rapidly shift chronic depression; electrotherapy units that can alleviate pain without side effects; combinations of complementary techniques that have been proven to dramatically improve cancer; subtle energy measurement devices that accurately pinpoint energy patterns before a disease ever becomes apparent in the body. Foreshadowing the engagement of the body's innate healing resources by electromagnetic healing, Thomas Edison exclaimed, more than a century ago, "The doctor of the future will give no medicine."[7] Yesterday's miracles become today's science.

Allopathic doctors will continue to hold an honored place in the pantheon of healers. But they will work side by side, on an equal professional footing, with many other healers. There might be a little old lady who looks like Mother Theresa, whose prayers have been discovered to work miracles, coming to visit patients daily. There might be an energetic, young, spiky-haired acupuncturist treating the patient expertly with needles, activating energy circuits that promote rapid regeneration. There may a professional crafter of visualizations and affirmations, a psychologist of the spirit who can formulate the exact combination of words and images that speak most powerfully to the subconscious mind of a particular patient. There may be an EFT practitioner in a lab coat, identifying and releasing layer after layer of inner wounding that has been impeding the patient's health. Nurses will be trained to guide a patient to the exact type of healer most likely to benefit their recovery. Indeed we predict that Nurse Practitioners will become primary providers of health care. Hospitals might start to look more like temples, filled with inspiring quotes, art, colors, and sounds, instead of cold, impersonal corridors."[8]

The pendulum has only begun its swing in the direction of soul medicine. The forces adding momentum to its movement are the exhaustion of the old system, its impossible costs, its inability to treat many systemic conditions, its lack of soul, and the enthusiasm of patients for soul medicine. We believe that, though the movement may look small today, treatment with soul medicine is a powerful trend that is rapidly transforming every current assumption about wellness. Our children will have an array of health options that we can only begin to imagine, and those that use soul medicine will be healthier as a result, despite the challenges of living on an overcrowded and overtaxed planet.

References

CH. 1 THE CONVERGENCE OF SPIRIT AND SCIENCE

1. Robins, Eric (2004). *The Heart of Healing* (Elite: Santa Rosa), p 281.
2. Barrett, Stephen (2003). A close look at naturopathy www.QuackWatch.org. Dec.
3. Lipton, Bruce (2005). *The Biology of Belief* (Elite: Santa Rosa), p 62.
4. *Science* (2001). Epigenetics special issue, 10 Aug, 293:5532.
5. Maret, K. (2005). Seven key challenges facing science. Fall, p 2.
6. Lipton, Bruce (2005) Quoted by Ardagh, Arjua, in *The Translucent Revolution* (Novato: New World Library), p 328.
7. Laslo, Ervin (1995). *The Whispering Pond: A Personal Guide to the Emerging Vision of Science* (Shaftesbury: Element Books).
8. Jeans, J. (1930). *The Mysterious Universe* (London: Longmans).
9. Lipton, Bruce (2005). Quoted by Ardagh, Arjua, in *The Translucent Revolution* (Novato: New World Library), p 341.
10. Oschman, James (2003). *Energy Medicine in Therapeutics and Human Performance* (Edinburgh: Butterworth Heineman), p 318.
11. McBride, J. L., Arthur, G., Brooks, R., Pilkington, L. (1998). The relationship between a patient's spirituality and health experiences. *Family Medicine.* Feb 30(2), p 122.
12. Powell, L. H., Shahabi, L., Thoresen, C. E. (2003). Religion and spirituality: linkages to physical health. *American Psychologist.* Jan 58(1), p 36.
13. Oxman, Thomas E., et al. (1995). Lack of social participation or religious strength and comfort as risk factors for death after cardiac surgery in the elderly. *Psychosomatic Medicine.* 57:5-15.
14. Schlitz, Marilyn (2005). The latest on prayer, touch and healing. *Spirituality and Health.* Nov/Dec p 35.
15. Dossey, Larry (1997). *Prayer is Good Medicine* (San Francisco: HarperSanFrancisco).
16. Dossey, Larry (2005). Non-local consciousness and the revolution in medicine in *Healing our Planet, Healing Our Selves* (Santa Rosa: Elite Books) p 153.
17. Institute of HearthMath (2003). *Emotional Energetics, Intuition and Epigenetics Research* (Boulder Creek: Institute of HearthMath), p 1.
18. Krucoff, Mitchell, and Crater, Suzanne (2001). Integrative noetic therapies as adjuncts to percutaneous intervention during unstable coronary syndromes. *American Heart Journal.* 142(5):760-769.
19. Ibid, McBride.
20. Borg, J., Andree, B., Soderstrom, H., Farde, L. (2003) The serotonin system and spiritual experiences. *American Journal of Psychiatry.* Nov; 160(11), p 1965.
21. Janowiak, J. J., Hackman, R. (1994). Meditation and college students' self-actualization and rated stress. *Psychological Reports.* Oct. 75(2), p 1007.
22. Doolittle, B. R., Farrell, M. (2004). The association between spirituality and depression in an urban clinic. *Journal of Clinical Psychiatry.* 6(3), p 114.
23. Koenig, H. G., George, L. K., Peterson, B. L. (1998). Use of health services by hospitalized medically ill depressed elderly patients. *American Journal of Psychiatry.* p 155:536-542.
24. Borg, J., Andree, B., *et. al.* (2004). The serotonin system and spiritual experiences. *American Journal of Psychiatry.* Sep; 161(9) 1720.
25. Koenig H. G., *et al.* (1997). *International Journal of Psychiatry in Medicine.* p 27:233-250.
26. Ibid, Krucoff.
27. Koenig, H. G., Larson, D. B. (1998). Use of hospital services, religious attendance, and religious affiliation. *Southern Medical Journal.* 91:925-932.

28. McSherry, E., Ciulla, M., Salisbury, S., Tsuang, D. (1987). *Social Compass*. 35(4):515-537.

29. Rowan, D. G., *et. al.* (1995). Self-actualization and empathy as predictors of marital satisfaction. *Psychological Reports*. Dec. 77(3-1):1011-6.

30. Koenig, H. G., *et al.* (1998). The relationship between religious activities and cigarette smoking in older adults. *Journal of Gerontology*. 53: 6.

31. Schmitt, R. R., Marx, D., VonDras, D. D. (2003). Spirituality as a moderator of alcohol use and attribution processes in college students. Paper presented at the Psi Chi Undergraduate Research Symposium at UW-Madison Apr 26.

32. Kark, J. D., et al. (1996). *American Journal of Public Health*. 86:341-346.

33. Daaleman, T. P., Perera, S., Studenski, S. A. (2004). Religion, spirituality, and health status in geriatric outpatients. *Annals of Family Medicine*. Jan-Feb 2(1), p 49.

34. Oxman, T. E., Freeman, D. H., and Manheimer, E. D. (1995). *Psychosomatic Medicine*. 57:5-15.

35. Powell, L. H., Shahabi, L., Thoresen, C. E. (2003). Religion and spirituality: linkages to physical health. *American Psychologist*. Jan 58(1), p 36.

36. Strawbridge, W. J., *et al.* (1997). *American Journal of Public Health*. 87:957-961.

Ch. 2 The Blueprint of Perfect Health

1. Ibid, Lazlo.

2. Eddington, Arthur (1994). Quoted in Wald, George, The cosmology of life and mind in *New Metaphysical Foundations of Modern Science* (Sausalito: IONS), p 130.

3. Rumi, in Barks, Coleman (1995). *The Essential Rumi* (San Francisco: HarperSanFrancisco), p 278.

4. Keller, J. C. (2005). Sacred minds. *Science and Theology News*. Dec p 18.

5. Cerinara, Gina (1991). *Many Mansions* (New York: Signet Books), p 82.

6. Graham, H. (2001). *Soul Medicine* (Dublin: Newleaf) p 253.

Ch. 3 A Physician's Search for Sacred Healing

1. Nolen, William (1947). *Healing: A Doctor in Search of a Miracle* (New York: Ballantine).

2. Ibid.

Ch. 4 Magic Precedes Science

1. Gaugelin, Michael (1974). *The Cosmic Clocks* (New York: Avon).

2. Dossey, Larry (2001). *Healing Beyond the Body* (Boston: Shambhala), p 235.

Ch. 5 Outstanding Healers of Our Time

1. Quoted in Dossey, Larry (2001). *Healing Beyond the Body* (Boston: Shambhala), p 29.

2. Remen, R. N. (2005). Recapturing the soul of medicine, in *Consciousness & Healing* (St. Louis: Elsevier), p 446.

3. Dossey, Larry (2001). *Healing Beyond the Body* (Boston: Shambhala), p 26.

4. www.HarryEdwards.org.uk

5. Ibid.

6. Cerutti, E. (1975). *Olga Worrall: Mystic With Healing Hands* (New York: Harper).

7. Grof, S. (2005). Psychology of the future, in *Consciousness & Healing* (St. Louis: Elsevier), p 265.

8. Ibid, Cerutti.

9. Steven L. Fahrion, S. L., Wirkus, M., Pooley, P. (1992). EEG amplitude, brain mapping, & synchrony in & between a bioenergy practitioner & client during healing. *Bridges*. 3:1.

10. Spear, Deena (2003). *Ears of the Angels* (Carlsbad: Hay House).

11. Northrup, Christiane (2004). *Health Wisdom for Women*. Nov.

12. Randall-May, C. (1999). *Pray Together Now: How to Find or Form a Prayer Group* (Shaftesbury: Element).

13. John Sewell does not have a web site. He practices during the day, but receives messages on his voice mail at 706-677-4934. He recommends a visit in person.

14. Eden, D. (1998). *Energy Medicine* (New York: Tarcher).

15. www.innersource.net/energy_medicine/case_history_em.htm.

16. Campbell, Rod (1996). *Healing From Love* (Auckland: Awareness).

17. Cayce reading 167-1, M.24, 7/25/39

18. Cayce reading 257-249, M.49, 12/5/42

19. Cayce reading 1173-6, M.28, 1/14/36

20. Cayce reading 1173-7, M.28, 11/28/36

21. Cayce reading 281-24, Prayer Group Series, 6/29/35

22. Oschman, James (2000). *Energy Medicine* (London: Churchill Livingstone), p 107.

Ch. 6 Characteristics of a Master Healer

1. McCraty, R., Atkinson, M, and Tomasino, D. (2003). Modulation of dna conformation by heart-focused intention (Boulder Creek: Institute of HearthMath), p 1.

2. www.JohnOfGod.com.

3. http://abcnews.go.com/Health/Primetime/story?id=482292&page=1

4. www.JohnOfGod.com.

5. Bird, C., and Tompkins, P., *The Secret Life of Plants* (Harper, 1989).

6. www.heartmath.org/ihm-action/press-room.

7. Rein, G., Atkinson, M., McCraty, R. (1995). The physiological and psychological effects of compassion and anger. *Journal of Advancement in Medicine.* 8(2): 87-105.

8. Ibid, hearthmath web site.

9. Krivorotov, V. (1987). Love therapy: a Soviet insight, in *The Heart of the Healer* (New York: Aslan), p 138.

10. Sha, Z. (2006). *Living Divine Relationships* (San Francisco: Heaven's Library), p 46.

11. Ibid, hearthmath web site.

12. Church, D. (2004). *The Heart of Healing* (Santa Rosa: Elite), p 31.

13. Sha, Z. (2006). *Healing the Heart of the World* (Santa Rosa; Elite), p 109.

14. Matthew 17:18, King James Version.

15. John 14:10, King James Version.

16. Langevin, M. (2006). *Healing the Heart of the World* (Santa Rosa; Elite), p 273.

17. Personal communication to author.

18. Bailey, Alice (1999). *Esoteric Healing* (New York: Lucis).

19. Personal communication to author. Dr. Nunley's Inner Counselor course is based on the work of Carl Jung, Abraham Maslow, and Robert Assagioli, and can be found at www.InnerCounselor.com.

20. Quoted in *Utne Reader* web site: http://www.utne.com/cgi-bin/udt/im.display.printable?client.id=utne_web_specials&story.id=616.

21. Grauds, C. (2006). The indigenous heart, in *Healing the Heart of the World* (Santa Rosa: Elite), p 232.

22. Ibid, *Utne.*

Ch 7 Soul, Mind and Medicine in History

1. Cruze, John Cerroll (1947). *The Incorruptibles* (Rockford: Tan).

2. James, William (1936). *The Varieties of Religious Experience* (New York: Modern Library). All quotes in this section are from pages 77-124.

3. *Random House College Dictionary,* (1984). (New York: Random House).

4. Dozor, Robert, (2004). *The Heart of Healing* (Elite: Santa Rosa), p 312.

Ch. 8 Re-Sacralyzing Healing

1. Motz, J. (1998). *Hands of Life: Use Your Body's Own Energy Medicine for Healing, Recovery and Transformation* (New York: Bantam), p 81.

2. Oz, M., and Roizen, M. F. (2005). *YOU: The Owner's Manual: An Insider's Guide to the Body that Will Make You Healthier and Younger* (New York: Collins).

Ch. 9 Sparking Spirit's Healing Flame

1. *Newsweek* (2003), Nov 12.

2. *Time* (1996), Jun 24.

3. *USA Weekend* (1997), Apr.

4. Barnes, P. M., Powell-Griner, E., McFann, K., Nahin, R. L. (2004). Complementary and alternative medicine use among adults: United States, 2002. *CDC Advance Data Report #343,* in NIH *Focus on Complementary and Alternative Medicine.* Volume XII, Number 1, Winter 2005.

5. Zhan, C., Miller, M. R. (2003). Excess length of stay, charges, and mortality attributable to medical injuries during hospitalization. *Journal of the American Medical Association.* Oct 8;290(14):1868-74.

6. Starfield, B. (2000). Is U.S. health really the best in the world? *Journal of the American Medical Association.* Jul 26:284(4):483-5.

7. www.garynull.com/documents/iatrogenic/deathbymedicine.htm.

8. Dossey, Larry (1996) *Prayer Is Good Medicine* (San Francisco: HarperSanFrancisco).

9. Ibid, Nolen.

10. Motluk, Alison (2005). 'Safe' painkiller is leading cause of liver failure. *New Scientist* 8. Dec 2529, p 19.

11. Vedantam, Shankar (2005). Study: new psychosis drugs no better than old ones. *Washington Post.* Sep 20.

12. Ibid, Vedantam.

13. Stein, R. and Kaufman, M. (2006).*Washington Post.* Jan 1.

14. Connor, Steve (2003). Glaxo chief: our drugs do not work on most patients. *Independent.* Dec 8.

15. Kelleher, Susan, and Wilson, Duff (2005). The hidden big business behind your doctor's diagnosis. *Seattle Times.* Jun 26.

16. Ibid, Kelleher.

17. Ingelfinger, Franz (1977). Health: a matter of statistics of feeling. *New England Journal of Medicine.* Feb 24, pp 448-49.

18. *New York Times* (2006). Seducing the medical profession. Feb 2.

19. Brennan, T. A., et al. (2006). Health industry practices that create conflicts of interest: A policy proposal for academic medical centers. *Journal of the American Medical Association.* 295:429-433.

20. Rubin, Rita (2006). Med schools urged to keep tabs on drugmakers. *USA Today.* Jan 24.

21. Osler, William (1943). *Aequanimitas* (Philadelphia: Blakeston).

22. Bernstein, R. K. (2003). *Dr. Bernstein's Diabetes Solution* (New York: Little, Brown).

23. Feinstein, D., *et. al.* (2005). *The Promise of Energy Psychology* (New York: Tarcher), p 14.

24. Gallo, F., and Vincenzi, H. (2000). *Energy Tapping* (Oakland: New Harbinger).

25. Craig, Gary. www.emofree.com.

26. Benor, Daniel. www.wholistichealingresearch.com/References/MBTs.asp.

27. Shealy, C. N., Thomlinson, R. P., Cox, R. H. and Borgmeyer, V. (1998). Osteoarthritis pain: A comparison of homeopathy and acetaminophen. *American Journal of Pain Management*. Vol. 8, No. 3, Jul pp 89-91.
28. Ibid, Ornish.

CH. 10 YOUR PERSONAL SOUL CONNECTION INVENTORY

1. Underhill, Evelyn (1993). *The Spiritual Life* (New York: Penguin).
2. Fillmore, Charles (1941). *The Twelve Powers of Man* (Missouri: Unity, sixth edition).
3. Ornish, Dean, ibid.
4. Here are the categories into which the questions fall:

1. FAITH

1. All things work together for good.
2. God is benevolent.
3. I have a soul that survives death.
4. My life on Earth is meaningful.

2. SERENITY, AND BEING IN THE MOMENT

5. Once a week or more, I reverently watch a sunset, sunrise, or natural scene.
6. I meditate, pray, or think about the beauty of life regularly.
7. I feel calm and serene when things go wrong.
8. I can face whatever life offers.

3. REASON, HONESTY, WISDOM AND UNDERSTANDING

9. I have sometimes wronged or harmed others.
10. I have apologized when I've wronged others.
11. I can learn from my problems and mistakes.
12. I am wise enough to make the right choices.
13. My spiritual beliefs change as I understand more.
14. I set reasonable standards and goals for myself.
15. During the course of my life, I have read three or more books about a religion other than my own.

4. LOVE, COMPASSION AND CHARITY

16. I helped someone within the last week.
17. Service to others equals service to God.
18. I tithe regularly.
19. In the last year, I have contributed to help others in misfortune.
20. When I see a person or animal in pain, I feel that pain.
21. I am connected to all living beings.
22. I go out of my way to help other people.

5. HOPE AND GRACE

23. Tomorrow will be better.
24. Miracles happen.
25. Human beings can change their ways and improve themselves.

6. FORGIVENESS

26. I usually forget wrongs that have been done to me within a few days.
27. I send blessings to people who have wronged me.
28. I send myself love when I've done something I wish I hadn't.

7. Tolerance and Non-Reactiveness

29. When I hear a belief that differs from mine, I consider it deeply.
30. I defend the right of others to have their beliefs, different from my own.
31. Religions other than mine may contain wisdom for me.
32. When someone acts badly towards me, I try and see their point of view.
33. When I become frustrated, I pause and calm myself.

8. Motivation, Will and Confidence

34. I can accomplish anything to which I apply myself.
35. I am able to keep focused even when other people don't believe in me.

9. Consistency and Application

36. I have a consistent daily spiritual practice.
37. I read religious or inspirational materials at least once a week.
38. I pray once a week or more for myself and others.
39. I believe that my attitude each day is more important than attending church.
40. I sent a blessing in my thoughts to someone else in the last two weeks.

10. Community

41. I have a trusted spiritual advisor.
42. I have two or more close friends.
43. I worship weekly at a church or spiritual center.
44. I said "I love you" to two or more people in the last week.
45. I gave someone an unexpected gift in the last month.

11. Joy

46. I often spontaneously feel great joy in my life.
47. I deliberately look for things to be happy about each day.

12. Gratitude

48. Every morning I'm thankful just to wake up.
49. I give thanks to God whenever good things happen.
50. I give thanks go God whenever bad things happen, even though I may not understand why.

Ch. 11 Soul Medicine as Primary Care

1. Szent-Gyorgi, Albert, quoted in Oschman, p 33.
2. Benson, H., McCallie, D. F. (1979). Angina pectoris and the placebo effect. *New England Journal of Medicine*. 300(25): 1424-9 13.
3. Moseley, J. B., *et. al.* (2002). A controlled trial of arthroscopic surgery for osteoarthritis of the knee. *New England Journal of Medicine*. Jul 11. 347:81-88.
4. Baylor College of Medicine Press Release. www.eurekalert.org/pub_releases/2002-07/bcom-sfc070802.php.
5. Eskenazi, L. (2005). Transformational surgery, in *Consciousness & Healing* (St. Louis: Elsevier), p 123.

6. Graham, H. (2001). *Soul Medicine* (Dublin: Newleaf), p 245.

7. Fetissov, S. (2005). *Proceedings of the National Academy of Sciences,* quoted in *The Economist.* Oct 1, p 75.

8. Marchione, M. (2005). Cancer survival tied to tumor size. Associated Press, Aug 7.

9. Schlitz, Marilyn (2005). The latest on prayer, touch and healing, in *Spirituality and Health.* Nov/Dec p 35.

10. Baltimore Sun (1999). Summarized at www.mcmanweb.com/article-18.htm.

11. Kirsch, I., and Sapirstein, G. (1998). Listening to Prozac but hearing placebo: A meta-analysis of antidepressant medication. *Prevention & Treatment.* Jun Vol 1(1) 2 [Article A].

12. Ibid, Kirsch.

13. Moore, T. J. (1999). No prescription for happiness. *Boston Globe.* Oct 17.

14. Kirsch, I, *et. al.* (2002). The emperor's new drugs: An analysis of antidepressant medication data submitted to the U.S. Food and Drug Administration. *Prevention & Treatment.* Jul Vol 5(23) 2.

Ch. 12 A Quantum Brain in a Neuroplastic Universe

1. Motluk, Alison (2005). Placebos trigger an opioid hit in the brain. *New Scientist.* 22:00 23 Aug.

2. Whitehouse, David (2003). Fake alcohol can make you tipsy. Summary of article in *Psychological Science,* reported in *BBC News.* Jul 1.

3. Penfield W., Baldwin M. (1952). Temporal lobe seizures and the technique of subtotal temporal lobectomy. *Annals of Surgery.* 136: 625-634.

4. Penrose, Roger (2002). *The Emperor's New Mind* (Oxford: Oxford University).

5. Damasio, Antonio (1994). *Descartes' Error: Emotion, Reason and the Human Brain* (New York: Grosset Putnam).

6. Summarized by Blakeslee, Sandra (2005). Hypnosis can profoundly change the brain. *New York Times.* Nov 22.

7. Ibid, Blakeslee.

8. Twain, Mark (1889). *A Connecticut Yankee in King Arthur's Court* (New York: Webster).

9. *Science* (2003). Brain maps perceptions, not reality. Nov 4.

Ch. 13 The Bodymind Electric

1. Ibid, Oschman, p 332.

2. Ibid, Oschman, p 8.

3. www.geocities.com/bioelectrochemistry/reymond.htm.

4. Ibid, reymond.htm.

5. Davydov. A. S. (1987). Excitons and solitons in molecular systems. *International Review of Cytology.* vol 106, pp 183-225.

6. Oschman, J. (2005). The intelligent body. *Bridges.* Spring 16:1 p 14.

7. Ibid, Davydov.

8. Becker, Robert O., & Selden, Gary (1985). *The Body Electric: Electromagnetism in the Foundation of Life* (New York: Morrow).

9. Ibid, Becker.

10. Maret, K. (2005). Seven key challenges facing science. *Bridges.* Spring 16:1 p 7.

11. Ibid, Becker.

12. *Alternative Medicine* (2002). High technology meets ancient medicine. Mar, p 93.

13. Ibid, *Alternative Medicine.*

14. Spence, Graham (2002). Quoted in Donna Eden, *Energy Medicine* (New York, Bantam), p 299.

15. There are many scientific references on Dr. Bonlie's web site, www.magneticosleep.com.

16. Ho, Mae-Wan, quoted in Oschman, p 310.

17. Shealy, 1993.

18. Reich, Wilhelm (1982). *The Bioelectric Investigation of Sexuality and Anxiety* (New York: Farrar, Straus, and Giroux).

19. Ibid.

20. Burr, H. S. (1957). Harold Saxton Burr. *Yale Journal of Biology & Medicine*. Vol 30. pp 161-167.

21. Ibid, Oschman, p 270.

22. Ibid, Oschman, p 62.

23. Ibid, Oschman, p 76.

24. Junnilia, S. Y. (1982). Acupuncture superior to piroxican in the treatment of osteoarthrosis. *American Journal Acupuncture*. Vol. 10, No. 4, Oct-Dec pp 341-346.

25. Helms, J. M. (1987). Acupuncture for the management of primary dysmenorrhea. *Obstetrics and Gynecology* Vol. 69, No. 1, Jan pp 51-56.

26. Shealy, C. N., Helms, J, McDaniels, A. (1990). Treament of male infertility with acupuncture. *The Journal of Neurological and Orthopaedic Medicine and Surgery*, Dec. Vol. 11, Issue 4, pp 285-86.

27. Hanson, P. E., Hansen, J. H. (1985). Acupuncture treatment of chronic tension headache—a controlled cross-over trial. *Cephalgia*. Vol. 5, No. 3, Sep pp 137-142.

28. Ballegaard, S., et al: Acupuncture in severestable angina pectoris—a randomized trial. Medical Dept. P. Rigshospitalet, University of Copenhagen, Denmark. *Acta. Med Scand*. Vol. 220, No. 4, pp 307-313.

29. Ibid, Oschman, p 266.

30. Wells, Steven, et al. (2003). Evaluation of a meridian-based intervention, emotional freedom techniques (EFT), for reducing specific phobias of small animals. *Journal of Clinical Psychology*, 59 (9), 943-966.

31. Ibid, Oschman, p 334.

CH. 14 SHIFTING THE PAIN PARADIGM

1. Shealy, C. N., Mortimer, J. T. and Reswick, J. B. (1967). Electrical inhibition of pain by dorsal column stimulation: Preliminary clinical report. *Anesthesia and Analgesia Current Researchers*. 46, pp 489-491.

CH. 15 UNZIPPING CHRONIC AND AUTOIMMUNE CONDITIONS

1. Selye, H. (1974). *The Stress of My Life: A Scientist's Memoirs* (New York: Van Nostrand Reinhold).

2. Benson, Herbert (2002). Interview entitled "Spirituality and Healing in Medicine" Ivanhoe Broadcast News Interview Transcript, Feb 4.

3. Snyderman, Ralph (2005). Creating a culture of health. *Spirituality and Health*. Dec, p 46.

4. Villoldo, Alberto (2000). *Shaman, Healer, Sage* (New York: Harmony) p 49.

5. Laslo, Ervin (1995). *The Whispering Pond: A Personal Guide to the Emerging Vision of Science* (Shaftesbury: Element Books).

6. Collinge, William (1998). *Subtle Energy* (New York: Warner), p 136.

CH. 16 HOW TO FIND YOUR IDEAL PRACTITIONER

1. Sha, Z. (2006). *Healing the Heart of the World* (Santa Rosa: Elite), p 109.

2. Benor, Daniel (1994). http://www.WholisticHealingResearch.com/Articles/IntuitAssessOverv.htm

3. Shealy, C. Norman (1996). *Ninety Days to Stress-Free Living* (London: Vega).

4. 2 Kings 5: 10-14.

CH. 17 MAINSTREAMING SOUL MEDICINE

1. Snyderman, Ralph (2005). Creating a culture of health, in *Spirituality and Health*. Dec p 46.

2. Quoted by Kristof, Nicholas (2006). Leading the fight against obesity. *New York Times*. Jan 31.

3. Moss, R. W. (2004). *The Moss Reports*. #127 Apr 4.

4. Smith, R. (1991). The poverty of medical evidence. *British Medical Journal*. 303, 5 Oct.

5. Hildenbrand, G. L. et al. (1995). Five-year survival rates of melanoma patients treated by diet therapy after the manner of Gerson: A retrospective review. *Alternative Therapies*. Sep 1(4): 29-37.

6. All three summarized on www.oohoi.com/inner_self/spiritual-healing

7. Nicholas H., Oberlies, N. H., Croy, V. L., *et. al.* (1997). The Annonaceous acetogenin bullatacin is cytotoxic against multidrug-resistant human mammary adenocarcinoma cells. *Cancer Letters* *115*. p 73-79.

8. Hirschberg, C. (2005). Living With Cancer *Consciousness & Healing* (St. Louis: Elsevier), p 163.

9. Washington Business Group on Health & Watson Wyatt Worldwide (2003). Creating a sustainable health care program. Eighth annual Washington Business Group on Health *Watson Wyatt Survey Report*.

10. Stewart, W. (2003). Lost productive time and cost due to common pain conditions in the US workforce. *Journal of the American Medical Association*. 290:2443-2454

11. Disease Management Congress (2003). *Employer Summit Highlights*. Sep 29-30; San Diego, California.

12. McCarberg, B., Wolf, J. (1999). Chronic pain management in a health maintenance organization. *The Clinical Journal of Pain*. 15:50-57.

13. BBC News (2000). *Health*. Feb 2.

14. Colllinge, W. (1996). *The American Holistic Health Association Complete Guide to Alternative Medicine* (New York: Warner), p 31.

15. Wirth, D. (1990). The effect of non-contact therapeutic touch on the healing rate of full thickness dermal wounds. *Subtle Energies*. 1(1), p 1-20.

16. Herman, P. M., Craig, B. M., Caspi, O. (2005). Is complementary and alternative medicine (CAM) cost-effective? a systematic review. *Complementary and Alternative Medicine*. 5:11 10.1186/1472-6882-5-11.

17. Dossey, Larry. (2001). *Healing Beyond the Body* (Boston: Shambhala), p 242.

18. McKeown, T., Brown, R. G. (1962) Reasons for the decline in mortality in England and Wales during the nineteenth century. *Population Studies*. 16:94-122.

19. http://www.ama-assn.org/ama/pub/category/12982.html

20. Keating, J. (1998). Chiropractic's quiet man. *Dynamic Chiropractic*. May 31, 16:12.

21. Loviglio, J. (2005). More traditional medical schools are including complementary and alternative medicine. Associated Press. Jun 5.

Ch. 18 Soul: Medicine of the Future

1. Oschman, James (2000). *Energy Medicine* (London: Churchill Livingstone), p 255.

2. Plante, L. (2005). Spirituality soars among scientists, study says. *Spirituality & Health*. Nov 2.

3. Janisse, T. (2005). Through conventional medicine to integral medicine *Consciousness & Healing* (St. Louis: Elsevier), p 461.

4. Jewish Theological Seminary (2004). Survey of physicians' views on miracles. (New York: Jewish Theological Seminary). www.jtsa.edu/research/finkelstein/surveys.

5. Woodcock, Alexander, & Davis, Monte (1978). *Catastrophe Theory* (New York: Viking Penguin), 9, quoted in Miller, William, 71.

6. Barnes, P. M., Powell-Griner, E., McFann, K., Nahin, R. L. (2004). Complementary and alternative medicine use among adults: United States, 2002. *CDC Advance Data Report #343,* in NIH *Focus on Complementary and Alternative Medicine*. Volume XII, Number 1, Winter 2005.

7. Edison, Thomas, quoted in Wayne, Michael (2005). *Quantum-Integral Medicine* (Saratoga Springs: iThink), p 159.

8. Gordon, J. (2005). The white house commission on CAM policy, in *Consciousness & Healing* (St. Louis: Elsevier), p 493.

Index

German Physical Society,
197
Giga-energy, 208
GigaTENS devices, 227
Gilbert, William, 195
Gordon, James, 274
Gordon, Richard, 76–77
Gospel of Relaxation, 121
Grad, Bernard, 64
Graham, Helen, 38, 174
Grauds, Constance, 105
Gray, Stephen, 196
Great Soul, infinite knowl-
edge of, 35
Green, Alyce, 63
Green, Elmer, 63, 65, 79,
168
Grof, Stanislav, 87–88
Guo, Zhi Chen, 100, 248
Gutiérrez, Diego, 20–21

H
Hagfors, Norman, 223
Hahnemann, Samuel, 144,
169, 215
Hales, Stephen, 196
Hands of Life (Motz), 126
Harris, Gardiner, 139
Harry Edwards Spiritual
Healing Sanctuary,
63
Harvey, William, 195
Haynes, George, 262
healer, healing the, 76
healers, spiritual
characteristics of, 36, 71,
87, 92
intention of, 92–96
partnership with, 250–251
qualifications of, 62
self-perception of, 91
spiritual practice of, 92,
96–97
healing. See holistic healing; spiritual heal-
ing
Healing: A Doctor in
Search of a Miracle
(Nolen), 44, 137
Healing Beyond the Body
(Dossey), 54

healing powers, transfer
of, 100
healing spas, 113–114
Healing Spirits (Joslow-
Rodewald, West-
Barker), 64
Healing the Heart of the
World (Grauds),
105
healing wisdom, access
to, 35
health
blueprint for, 34
community and, 155
as dynamic process, 38
foundation for, 47
soul connection and, 29–30
heart
DNA structure change and
coherence of, 18–20
early concepts of, 126–127
emotional states and rate
variability of, 91–92
intention and congruence
of, 96
The Heart of Healing
(Church), 53, 99
The Heart of the Healer
(Church), 53
Heartmath Institute, 92,
190
Hippocrates, 126–129
Hippocratic Oath, 127–128
Ho, Mae-Wan, 208–209
Hodgkin, A.L., 199
holistic healing. See also
spiritual healing
conflict between allopathic
and, 169
cost of society's ignorance
of, 257–260
electromagnetic characteristics of, 229–230
first point of intervention
of, 20
nature of true, 38, 85
safe/non-invasive, 38–39
surgery and, 20
therapies, types of, 17, 37–39
holistic healing movement,
154

holistic practitioners, finding, 245–252
Holmes, Ernest, 116
Holos University Graduate
Seminary, 46, 103,
107, 263
holy epiphanies, 115
homeopathy, 144, 169–170
Houston, Jean, 104
Huckabee, Mike, 255
human beings
individuation of, 154
limited personality nature
of, 148–149
microsmic nature of, 34
soul nature of, 148–149
human bodies
electromagnetic framework
of, 235, 239
as energy systems, 31–32,
37–38, 212
humors of, 127
meridians of, 213–219
semiconductive capabilities
of, 214
human genome project, 14
Human Unity Conference,
52–53
humanistic psychology
movement, 154
Huxley, A.F., 199

I
iatrogenic illnesses, 136
illness. See disease/illness
Immunoglobulin-A, 95–96
information, holographic
storage of, 190
Ingelfinger, Franz, 139
Inner Counselor, 103
Institute of Heartmath
(California), 18
Integrative Medical Clinic
(California), 122–123
integrative medicine. See
spiritual healing
intention, effects of, 18–19,
35–36, 96
International Council
of Magnetic
Therapists, 206
intuitive diagnosis, 77